Podcasting for Medical Professionals

Joanna Parga-Belinkie • Katie Lockwood
Tony Tarchichi
Editors

Podcasting for Medical Professionals

Taking a Medical Podcast from Idea to Recording and Reality

Springer

Editors
Joanna Parga-Belinkie
Division of Neonatology
Children's Hospital of Philadelphia
Philadelphia, PA, USA

Katie Lockwood
Department of General Pediatrics
Children's Hospital of Philadelphia
Philadelphia, PA, USA

Tony Tarchichi
Pediatric Hospital Medicine
Children's Hospital of Pittsburgh
Pittsburgh, PA, USA

ISBN 978-3-032-16479-7 ISBN 978-3-032-16480-3 (eBook)
https://doi.org/10.1007/978-3-032-16480-3

This Springer imprint is published by the registered company Springer Nature Switzerland AG
The registered company address is: Gewerbestrasse 11, 6330 Cham, Switzerland

Contents

Chapter 1
The Evolution of Medical Podcasts: Tracing History and Looking Ahead

Michael D. Patrick Jr

Introduction to Medical Podcasting

In recent years, medical podcasting has emerged as an innovative and influential medium for disseminating health-related information. Medical podcasts provide accessible, engaging content for various audiences, including healthcare professionals, medical students, patients, and the general public. Podcasts encompass a broad range of topics, from clinical education and patient narratives to the latest research updates, making them an invaluable resource for staying informed in a fast-paced and constantly evolving field.

The convenience and accessibility of podcasts are key factors in their widespread appeal. Unlike traditional educational materials that require visual engagement, podcasts allow listeners to absorb information while on the go—whether commuting, exercising, or completing daily tasks. This flexibility makes medical podcasts a practical solution for busy professionals who may struggle to find time for continued education in their demanding schedules [1]. Furthermore, the audio format allows for a more personal connection with the content, often enhanced by hosts who bring a relatable, conversational tone to complex medical topics.

Medical podcasts have also proven to be a powerful tool for filling gaps in traditional medical education. By offering easily accessible content that covers a wide range of subjects, podcasts support a more holistic learning experience. They also provide insights into areas that might be underrepresented in formal curricula, such as patient perspectives and interdisciplinary approaches to care. This complements more structured learning by providing real-world context and fostering a deeper understanding of healthcare challenges and innovations.

M. D. Patrick Jr (✉)
Nationwide Children's Hospital, The Ohio State University College of Medicine, Columbus, OH, USA
e-mail: michael.patrick@nationwidechildrens.org

J. Parga-Belinkie et al. (eds.), *Podcasting for Medical Professionals*,
https://doi.org/10.1007/978-3-032-16480-3_1

The reach and impact of medical podcasts extend beyond healthcare professionals. With topics that often resonate with the general public, these podcasts also play a crucial role in patient education and public health advocacy. For example, podcasts covering mental health topics have empowered listeners to seek help and better understand conditions that are often stigmatized [2]. Similarly, podcasts featuring patient stories can promote empathy and enhance the patient-provider relationship by providing healthcare professionals with insights into the patient experience.

Over the past decade, medical podcasts have transformed how information is shared within the healthcare community. Notable examples include *The Curbsiders Internal Medicine Podcast*, *Flip the Script*, *The Clinical Problem Solvers*, *2 Docs Talk*, and the *Key Literature in Medical Education (KeyLIME) Podcast* [3]. These shows not only share valuable knowledge but also foster a sense of community among listeners, connecting healthcare professionals and laypeople alike with informative and engaging content.

The versatility and impact of medical podcasts underscore their value in today's healthcare landscape. As the field evolves, podcasts will likely play an even more significant role in medical education and patient communication. By providing accessible and engaging content, medical podcasts have become an essential tool for healthcare professionals and the public, enhancing how medical information is disseminated and understood.

The Origins of Podcasts

The origins of podcasting can be traced back to early audio formats and precursors, such as radio broadcasts and audio blogs. Radio shows had long provided serialized audio content, but it was not until the advent of digital technology that on-demand audio became a reality. In the 1990s, as the internet grew, audio blogging emerged as one of the first steps toward what would become podcasting. Innovators in the tech world began exploring ways to distribute audio content online, setting the stage for podcasts as we know them today [4].

The term "podcast" itself was coined in 2004 by journalist Ben Hammersley, who combined the words "iPod" and "broadcast" to describe this new form of media. However, the groundwork for podcasting was laid by two key figures: Dave Winer, a software developer, and Adam Curry, a former MTV video jockey. Winer developed the RSS feed with an enclosure tag, which allowed audio files to be distributed automatically to users. Curry used this technology to create the first true podcast, a show called *Daily Source Code*, which became the prototype for future podcasts [5].

Apple's iPod played a crucial role in the popularization of podcasts. The device's portability allowed users to take audio content with them, and the subsequent integration of podcasts into iTunes in 2005 provided a seamless platform for discovering and downloading podcasts. This development was transformative, making podcasts more accessible and significantly boosting their popularity [6]. Apple continued to shape the podcasting landscape by providing a centralized directory that helped listeners find and follow shows. As smartphone technology advanced, dedicated podcast apps emerged, further increasing podcast accessibility and driving a new wave of growth [7].

Podcasting quickly moved from a niche medium to a mainstream platform. By the late 2000s, podcasts were being produced on a vast range of topics, from entertainment and news to education and specialized fields such as medicine. Early medical podcasts, like *EMCrit* and *The Dr. Axe Show*, demonstrated the potential of podcasts as educational tools, particularly for healthcare professionals who needed access to information on the go. These podcasts provided timely insights and discussions on medical topics, contributing to the medium's growing credibility as a source of professional knowledge.

The Following Timeline Highlights Some Key Events in the Early Evolution of Podcasting

- 1993: First known audio blogs appear as early forms of digital audio content sharing.
- 2000: Dave Winer introduces the RSS feed with enclosure tags, enabling the distribution of audio files.
- 2004: The term "podcast" is coined, and *Daily Source Code* is launched, marking the start of modern podcasting.
- 2005: Apple adds podcasting support to iTunes, making podcasts easily discoverable and downloadable.
- 2010: The rise of smartphones and dedicated podcast apps expands the audience, propelling podcasts into the mainstream.

Today, podcasting continues to evolve with the advent of new formats, monetization models, and a widening audience base. The growth of podcasts in healthcare specifically underscores their utility in professional education, patient communication, and public health advocacy. Podcasts now play a vital role in how information is shared across the medical community, paving the way for even more innovative uses in the years to come. [8].

An Opportunity for Digital Storytelling

Digital storytelling has become essential for engaging audiences, particularly in medical podcasting. It combines narrative techniques with digital media to convey information in a way that is both relatable and impactful. In the context of medical podcasts, digital storytelling brings medical concepts to life, making them more accessible and understandable for a broad audience, including healthcare professionals, students, and laypeople alike [9].

At its core, compelling storytelling in digital media relies on several key elements. The first is a compelling narrative structure, typically including a beginning that establishes context, a middle that introduces challenges or conflicts, and a resolution that offers insights or takeaways. This structure helps to engage the audience by creating a natural flow that holds their attention and keeps them invested in the story. Authenticity is another crucial component, as it builds trust with listeners. In medical storytelling, authenticity often stems from using real-life examples and drawing from personal experiences, which fosters a connection with the audience and lends credibility to the content.

Emotion plays a significant role in storytelling, especially in medical contexts with highly sensitive and complex topics. By appealing to emotions, storytellers can foster empathy and help listeners connect on a personal level [10]. This is particularly important in medical podcasting, where the subject matter often involves human suffering, resilience, and healing. A well-told story can evoke a range of emotions, from hope to curiosity to compassion, helping listeners to engage with and remember the information presented.

The role of voice, tone, and pacing cannot be overstated in digital storytelling. In podcasts, the spoken word is the primary vehicle for conveying emotion and tone, significantly affecting how the audience perceives the content. A calm, reassuring voice can make listeners feel comfortable and open to learning, while a dynamic and passionate tone can energize and inspire them. Proper pacing ensures the story unfolds at a rate that keeps listeners engaged without overwhelming them, allowing complex medical concepts to be presented in a digestible manner.

In medicine, storytelling is a powerful means to humanize complex medical topics. For example, a medical podcast might share a patient's journey through diagnosis, treatment, and recovery, illustrating not only the clinical aspects of the condition but also the personal experiences accompanying it. This approach allows listeners to see beyond the symptoms and procedures to understand the patient as a whole person. Such storytelling fosters empathy among healthcare professionals and enriches their perspective on patient care [11].

Storytelling enhances listeners' retention of complex information by providing context and emotional resonance. When facts are embedded within a story, they become more memorable and meaningful. This is particularly beneficial in medical education, where students and professionals must retain vast amounts of information. Storytelling can also promote reflective practice, as listeners relate the stories they hear to their own experiences and consider how they might apply the lessons learned in their practice.

Digital storytelling, therefore, is not merely a means of sharing information—it is a transformative tool that brings medicine's humanity to the forefront. By combining narrative structure, emotional resonance, and an authentic voice, medical podcasts can communicate complex ideas that resonate with and inspire their listeners.

Prevalence and Demographics of Podcast Listeners

The podcasting landscape has experienced tremendous growth over the past two decades, transforming from an amateur medium to a mainstream phenomenon. As of 2024, over four million podcasts are available, covering diverse topics and attracting a vast audience. This growth reflects the increasing desire for on-demand audio content, with the total number of podcast listeners worldwide expected to reach over 600 million by 2026. This expansion has been fueled by the proliferation of mobile devices and streaming platforms, which have made accessing podcasts more effortless than ever before [12].

According to Edison Research, 59% of Americans between the ages of 12 and 34, 55% between the ages of 35 and 55, and 27% of those 55 and older have listened to a podcast in the past month. This broad distribution highlights podcasting's appeal across different age groups. Gender representation is nearly balanced, with men (51%) slightly more likely to listen to podcasts than women (48%) [13].

The popularity of medical podcasts has mirrored this overall growth, attracting healthcare professionals, medical students, and the general public. Medical podcasts are particularly valued for their accessibility and convenience, providing busy professionals with opportunities for learning and professional development during their daily routines. Recent data suggests that 81% of healthcare professionals and 55% of the general public listen to medical podcasts. This ability to access medical information on demand has been a game-changer for both education and patient engagement [14].

Listening habits provide further insight into podcast consumption. On average, podcast listeners engage with eight episodes per week, with 23% of listeners spending over 10 h per week listening to podcasts. Smartphones are the most popular device for podcast listening, with 70% of listeners choosing mobile apps for streaming or downloading content. Apple Podcasts and Spotify are the leading platforms, collectively capturing around 70% of the podcast audience. Other popular platforms include YouTube, Amazon Music, Audible, iHeartRadio, and various apps on iOS and Android [12].

The growing popularity of medical podcasts underscores their impact as an educational medium. They cater to a diverse audience, from students and professionals to patients, fostering a deeper understanding of complex medical topics. By combining accessibility, convenience, and engaging content, podcasts have become an indispensable tool in medical education and public health communication.

Use of Podcasts in Medical Education

Recently, podcasts have gained recognition as valuable educational tools within medical training. Their flexibility and accessibility allow students and healthcare professionals to learn on their own terms, providing opportunities for continuous education outside traditional classroom settings. Podcasts have proven especially beneficial in medical training by offering a convenient medium for staying updated with the latest medical knowledge, case studies, and expert insights [15].

One key advantage of using podcasts in medical training is their ability to enhance knowledge retention. Podcasts often incorporate storytelling and interviews with subject matter experts, which can make complex information more relatable and memorable. According to a study on learning preferences among medical students, podcasts improved information retention by presenting content in a conversational format that promotes active listening. This format allows listeners to engage with the material in a way that feels less formal yet highly informative, creating a learning experience that is both enjoyable and effective.

Podcasts also offer access to specialized content on demand. Unlike traditional lectures or seminars tied to specific schedules and locations, podcasts can be accessed anytime, anywhere, making them ideal for busy medical students and professionals. This flexibility supports continuous learning, as listeners can integrate podcasts into their daily routines, whether commuting, exercising, or taking breaks. Additionally, podcasts provide exposure to various perspectives, as they often feature diverse voices from various fields and specialties. This allows learners to explore topics outside their immediate areas of study, promoting a more well-rounded understanding of healthcare [16].

Several medical schools and residency programs have begun integrating podcasts into their curricula as supplementary learning tools. For example, some programs assign specific podcast episodes for students to listen to before or after lectures, creating opportunities for reflective learning and reinforcing key concepts. Podcasts focused on clinical updates, case studies, and interviews with healthcare leaders are particularly popular in these settings, as they provide insights into real-world medical practice and recent advancements in the field. Incorporating podcasts into formal education helps students develop critical skills for their future careers, such as critical thinking, empathy, and a commitment to lifelong learning [17].

However, while podcasts are valuable supplementary resources, they are not without challenges. One limitation is that they may not provide the same level of depth as traditional textbooks or lectures. Additionally, since anyone can create and distribute podcasts, the quality and accuracy of information can vary. Educators and learners must critically evaluate podcast content to ensure it aligns with evidence-based practices and is presented by credible sources [18]. Addressing these challenges requires a balanced approach, using podcasts with other educational resources to create a comprehensive learning experience.

Despite these considerations, podcasts have carved out a meaningful role in medical training by providing accessible, engaging, and relevant content that complements traditional educational methods. As the medical field continues to evolve, podcasts are likely to play an even more significant role in supporting the education of healthcare professionals, fostering a culture of continuous learning, and enhancing the overall quality of medical training [19].

Podcasts Across Medical Specialties

Medical podcasts have evolved to cater to a wide array of specialties, providing targeted content that addresses the unique needs and interests of professionals within specific fields. These podcasts offer valuable resources for current practitioners and those in training by focusing on specialty-specific topics. Specialty-specific podcasts cover various subjects, from clinical advancements and case studies to discussions on the latest research, tailored to the nuances of each field [20].

Podcasts in nearly thirty medical specialties and subspecialties, including internal medicine, pediatrics, surgery, and psychiatry, have garnered substantial followings as they deliver content directly relevant to healthcare professionals working within these areas. For example, in pediatrics, *PediaCast CME* offers insights into child health and wellness, covering topics like vaccination, pediatric obesity, and child development. These episodes provide updates on clinical practices and address broader issues related to child health, such as mental well-being and family dynamics, which are crucial for practitioners in this field [21].

In surgery, podcasts like *Behind the Knife* have become essential tools for surgical residents and practicing surgeons. This podcast delves into surgical techniques, case studies, and critical reflections on patient care. Its hosts, who are experienced surgeons, often invite guest experts to discuss complex surgical cases and share their insights on best practices. By offering deep dives into specialized topics, *Behind the Knife* supports a culture of continuous learning within the surgical community, where staying updated with new techniques and approaches is paramount [22].

Psychiatry-focused podcasts, such as *The Psych Central Show*, provide listeners with access to discussions on mental health, therapy techniques, and the latest research in psychological science. This podcast addresses clinical and public perspectives on mental health, making it useful for psychiatrists, therapists, and those interested in understanding mental health issues. Specialty-specific podcasts like these create spaces for professionals to explore topics relevant to their practice and stay informed about developments within their field, enhancing their ability to deliver effective care [23].

The benefits of specialty-specific podcasts extend beyond knowledge acquisition; they also help foster a sense of community among professionals who may otherwise have limited opportunities for interaction and discussion outside their workplace [24]. These podcasts allow listeners to engage with others who share their professional interests, promoting shared learning and camaraderie. Additionally, specialty podcasts provide a platform for discussing challenges unique to each field, such as the state of child healthcare in pediatrics, the technical complexities encountered in surgery, and ethical dilemmas faced in psychiatry. By addressing these specialized concerns, podcasts offer listeners a chance to reflect on their practice and consider new approaches to patient care.

Despite their many advantages, specialty-specific podcasts face challenges in maintaining relevance and depth, as content must be frequently updated to keep pace with advances in medical research and clinical practice. Moreover, given the rapid evolution of medical knowledge, these podcasts must balance the need for comprehensive coverage with the time constraints of their audiences. Looking to the future, there are opportunities for increased collaboration across specialties, where podcasters could create episodes that address interdisciplinary topics or bring together experts from various fields to discuss shared healthcare challenges.

In conclusion, specialty-specific podcasts provide an invaluable service to the medical community by offering targeted, relevant content that fosters ongoing learning and professional connection. As the medium continues to evolve, these podcasts will become even more integral to how medical professionals access and engage with specialized knowledge.

Call to Action

As you journey through this textbook, consider the immense potential of medical podcasts to shape healthcare education, practice, and patient engagement. Each chapter will delve into how to create, curate, and leverage podcast content to reach diverse audiences effectively. Whether you are a seasoned podcaster or new to this medium, explore how podcasts can enhance your role as a healthcare professional, educator, and advocate. Embrace the power of this dynamic platform to share knowledge, inspire change, and connect with others in the medical community.

References

1. Berk J, Trivedi SP, Watto M, Williams P, Centor R. Medical education podcasts: where we are and questions unanswered. J Gen Intern Med. 2020;35:2176–8.
2. Carrotte ER, Blanchard M, Groot C, Hopgood F, Phillips L. Podcasts, mental health, and stigma: exploring motivations, behaviors, and attitudes among listeners. Commun Stud. 2023;74(3):200–16.
3. Lomayesva NL, Martin AS, Dowley PA, Davies NW, Olyha SJ, Wijesekera TP. Five medical education podcasts you need to know. Yale J Biol Med. 2020;93(3):461–6.
4. Hoyt E, Morris JW. One. Podcast archaeology: researching proto-podcasts and early born-digital audio formats. In: Saving new sounds: podcast preservation and historiography. Ann Arbor: University of Michigan Press; 2021.
5. Bottomley AJ. Podcasting: a decade in the life of a "new" audio medium: introduction. J Radio Audio Media. 2015;22(2):164–9.
6. Berry R. A Golden Age of Podcasting? Evaluating Serial in the Context of Podcast Histories. Journal of Radio and Audio Media. 2015;22(2):170–8. ISSN 19376529.
7. Sullivan JL. The platforms of podcasting: past and present. Social media+ society. 2019;5(4):2056305119880002.
8. Kiernan MA, Mitchell BG, Russo PL. The power of podcasts: exploring the endless possibilities of audio education and information in medicine, healthcare epidemiology, and antimicrobial stewardship. Antimicrob Stewardship Healthcare Epidemiol. 2023;3(1):e98. https://doi.org/10.1017/ash.2023.178.

9. Stukus DR, Patrick MD, Nuss KE, Patrick MD. The art of digital storytelling. In: Social media for medical professionals: strategies for successfully engaging in an online world. Cham: Springer; 2019. p. 83–100.
10. Liao HC, Wang YH. Storytelling in medical education: narrative medicine as a resource for interdisciplinary collaboration. Int J Environ Res Public Health. 2020;17(4):1135.
11. Gray JB. The power of storytelling: using narrative in the healthcare context. J Commun Healthc. 2009;2(3):258–73.
12. Riverside. Podcast statistics and trends for 2025 (& why they matter). 2025. https://riverside.fm/blog/podcast-statistics. Accessed 25 Feb 2025.
13. Edison Research. The Podcast Consumer. 2024. https://www.edisonresearch.com/wp-content/uploads/2024/05/The-Podcast-Consumer-2024-Presentation.pdf. Accessed 25 Feb 2025.
14. Lee C, Zhou MS, Wang ER, Huber M, Lockwood KK, Parga J. Health care professional and caregiver attitudes toward and usage of medical podcasting: questionnaire study. JMIR Pediatrics Parenting. 2022;5(1):e29857.
15. Malecki SL, Quinn KL, Zilbert N, Razak F, Ginsburg S, Verma AA, Melvin L. Understanding the use and perceived impact of a medical podcast: qualitative study. JMIR Med Educ. 2019;5(2):e12901.
16. Hurst EJ. Podcasting in medical education and health care. J Hosp Librariansh. 2019;19(3):214–26.
17. Shrivastava SR, Shrivastava PS, Bankar NJ. Adoption of a comprehensive approach to streamline the integration of podcast-based learning in medical education. J Clin Sci. 2024;21(3):158–60.
18. Lin M, Thoma B, Trueger NS, Ankel F, Sherbino J, Chan T. Quality indicators for blogs and podcasts used in medical education: modified Delphi consensus recommendations by an international cohort of health professions educators. Postgrad Med J. 2015;91(1080):546–50.
19. Kelly JM, Perseghin A, Dow AW, Trivedi SP, Rodman A, Berk J. Learning through listening: a scoping review of podcast use in medical education. Acad Med. 2022;97(7):1079–85.
20. Caldwell KE, Zarate-Rodriguez JG, Fox JC, Yaeger L, Wise PE. Listen up: a systematic review of the utilization and efficacy of podcasts for medical education. Glob Surg Educ J Assoc Surg Educ. 2024;3(1):107.
21. PediaCast CME. PediaCast CME: a pediatric podcast for providers. 2025. https://www.pediacastcme.org/. Accessed 25 Feb 2025.
22. Behind the Knife. Behind the knife: podcast episodes. 2025. https://app.behindtheknife.org/home. Accessed 25 Feb 2025.
23. Psych Central. The Psych Central Podcast. 2025. https://psychcentral.com/authors/the-psych-central-podcast. Accessed 25 Feb 2025.
24. Miller KA, Keeney T, Fialkowski A, Srinivasan S, Singh TA, Kesselheim J, et al. Leveraging podcasts to introduce medical students to the broader community of health care professionals. MedEdPORTAL. 2021;17:11191.

Chapter 2
How and Why Podcasts Are Used in Medical Education

Michael Cosimini

Who Is Making Medical Education Podcasts and Why

Why Podcast in Medical Education

As you set out making a podcast let's consider some examples of who is making podcasts and why they are doing it. In this chapter podcasting associated with institutions and journals are highlighted; still projects are often the babies of individuals whose real purposes might not be fully reflected in the literature. Take for example *Febrile* which began as a med-peds infectious diseases(ID) fellow's project and has grown into a collection of resources sponsored by the Infectious Disease Society of America (IDSA). Described in the literature *Febrile* intends to "provide a free open-access educational resource with high-quality content about ID" as well as building community in ID, and inspiring the next generation of ID physicians [1]. In the first episode Dr. Dong goes farther and also describes her goal to share the joy of ID case conferences and to treasure her own med-peds identity [2].

In his book *Scholarly Podcasting* Ian Cook highlights some ideas for why scholars podcast. Based on interviews he describes podcasting as an insurgent act going against academic structures that hamper creativity, transformation, and generosity [3]. Table 2.1 summarizes some of these reasons. How do these fit with your own motives or goals for podcasting? Or which have you found along your podcasting path so far? Get out a highlighter and pick two.

M. Cosimini (✉)
Division of General Pediatrics, Oregon Health and Science University, Portland, OR, USA
e-mail: cosimini@ohsu.edu

J. Parga-Belinkie et al. (eds.), *Podcasting for Medical Professionals*,
https://doi.org/10.1007/978-3-032-16480-3_2

Table 2.1 Why people do scholarly podcasting from *Scholarly Podcasting* [3]

Creativity	Inspires innovation in pedagogy such as creating content for students or mentoring students in their own content creation Intimate, in how it is consumed and as a way that podcasters can express emotion that would not be present in written work Vulnerability which leads to opportunity to think through and improve ideas as opposed to presented complete work in a written form
Transformative	Freedom to work outside of the traditional academic channels Gaining skills and knowledge through the process of the work preparing the podcasts Rewarding in networking, self promotion, and in some cases recognition academically
Generosity	Opening scholarship to broader voices and the community Cultivating listenership through a feeling of togetherness Creation of communities around new voices

Who Is Making Medical Education Podcasts

Medical education podcasts come from a variety of sources including individuals or groups outside of institutions, universities, journals/professional groups as well as commercially produced podcasts. The field has matured over two decades [4] and the producers of this content, and the role of institutions have shifted. Podcasts in medical education are documented as early as 2005 with 42 podcasts in critical care and emergency medicine(EM) through 2013 [5]. Since 2013 the total number of active podcasts and blogs in critical care and EM surprisingly has declined [6] and there has been more uptake of institution sponsorship (44%), advertisement or other methods of financial support for the remaining sites.

So where are we today? A cross section listing 38 infectious disease podcasts as of 2024 shows the current breadth of the groups producing podcasts [7]. These include institutions, journals, professional societies, individually produced podcasts some of which were later sponsored by societies such as *ID:IOTS: Infectious Diseases Insight of Two Specialists* (started 2021 and later supported by the British Infection Association), and podcasts in an independent network such as MicrobeTV including *Infectious Disease Puscast*. Examples from this study are categorized by the groups producing the podcasts in Table 2.2.

Another study looking at the top 100 medical podcasts from 2018 to 2020 found that 51 were intended for physician audiences. Among these individuals (35.2%), companies (31.4%), and journals (23.5%) were the most common affiliations. Professional societies (5.9%), universities (2%), and residency programs (2%) were much less common [8]. These were clustered by specialty with physicians in EM (21%), Pediatrics (9.8%) and Internal Medicine (9.8%) being the most common single specialty audiences. Looking at top podcasts likely concentrates those fields for which the largest audiences are available. This is also worth keeping in mind as you review your metrics as a high impact pediatric rheumatology podcast may be the fraction the size of a modest EM podcast.

Table 2.2 Examples of infectious disease podcasts from Oehler et al. 2024 categorized by type of group publishing them

Group producing	Podcasts examples
Institutions	IDPodcasts—USF Division of Infectious Diseases Osterholm Update—University of Minnesota De-CIPHERing Infectious Disease—CIPhER—Center for Innovative Pharmacy Education & research University of North Carolina Chapel Hill
Professional societies and journals	Breakpoints—Society for Infectious Disease Pharmacists Editors in Conversation—American Society for Microbiology Journals Communicable—Clinical Microbiology and Infections Communications Let's Talk ID—Infectious Disease Society of America AJIC: Science Into Practice—Association for Professionals in Infection Control and Epidemiology
Individuals	Transplant ID Cast—Shmuel Shoham Transmissible: A Public Health Podcast—Jessica Stahl Lets meet the virologists—Larissa Thackray
Individuals with sponsorship	Febrile—Sara Dong—Infectious Disease Society of America ID:IOTS: Infectious Diseases Insight of Two Specialists—Jame McRae and Callum Mutch—British infectious association
Independent Networks	Infectious Disease Puscast—Microbe TV This Week in Microbiology—Microbe TV This Week in Virology—Microbe TV

Journal and Society Podcasts—Metrics, Dissemination, Translation and Community

Journals have had podcasts since early in the technology's history. A 2009 review of podcasts from journals describes podcasts available from eight of 100 general medical and internal medicine journals [9]. This included household names such as NEJM (since 2005) described as having a bit of an echo and being"dull", Lancet (2006), JAMA (2006), Annals of Internal Medicine (2007), and BMJ (2006). Early journal podcasts had formats including a reading of the journal's abstracts, author interviews and editor's comments [10]. Weekly interviews of an author of an "Interesting, informative and important" paper started in Neurology in 2007 and the history of this journal podcast highlights the role of a single motivated individual in a successful podcast even when published under the name of a journal. Listen to this reference for more on that [11].

Since the early days medical journal's podcasts have grown in number and quality with the early adopters NEJM, JAMA and Lancet now hosting numerous podcasts including the now classic NEJM single voice summarizing the issue format. Annals has doubled its offerings to two podcasts including one by the man the legend Bob (Centor criteria) Centor. Journal and society podcasts are getting bigger and more complex with time. For example Breakpoints, from the Society for Infectious Disease Pharmacists has a committee of about 40 members supporting its development [12].

What Do Journals Want to Gain from Social Media?

Social media editors have a variety of roles and responsibilities including branding, knowledge translation and dissemination. Dissemination is not just to the journal's typical audience but also the public, policymakers and the media [13]. Social media editors see one of their roles as communicating science and being a reliable source of information [14]. Interviews of social media editors found them largely focusing on reader engagement and dissemination [15]. They worked to highlight new and potentially interesting content with much of this done by posting or hosting dialog on social media, though more involved strategies were also described in these interviews. Here podcasts are one of many tools available in the domain of social media. Journals may aim to have podcasts improve journal metrics (article views, citations, impact factor) or be a channel to reach an audience that would not otherwise be reading the content from the journal [16]. Studies looking at the impact of social media use by journals typically report metrics of how people have interacted with the social media (views, engagement, reposting) and how this has impacted access of the articles (link clicks, pageviews, downloads) presuming that increasing the use of the journals material is the goal [17]. This is consistent with data on the content of posts on social media by medical journals who largely post to promote specific issues or articles [18] and with themes from social media editors perspective on the journal's goals as being engagement (readers, authors, public), branding and metrics [15].

Journals who explicitly provide the reasons for having podcasts often describe trying to make the content of the journals applicable to listeners. Academic Medicine uses the podcast to "support the professional development and academic success of learners and colleagues across the academic medicine career continuum [19]." Neurology's Podcast provides "Practical, relevant, timely information for neurologists and all clinicians to practice the best possible medicine for our patients." Centor's podcast Annals on Call aims to "discuss the implications of the articles" for listeners. Academic Pediatrics aims to, "connect listeners with the authors and editors of the journal and inform all of our clinical, educational, research and advocacy practice." This goal is informed by the social nature of social media and the idea that unidirectional broadcasting of content is not as effective in sustained engagement as building a community. Listeners to medical education podcasts do so in part to feel connected to a community [20] and podcasts are able to broaden and connect learning communities [21]. Supporting the social aspect, one randomized study showed broadcasting articles from a journal's social media account was not effective in increasing page views compared to control articles that were not promoted; however the addition of posts from individual editors did result in increased pageviews [22]. Other studies have also shown a lack of impact from posting articles from journal's social media accounts alone [23, 24].

Is Podcasting Effective to Bring Audiences to Journal Articles?

While there is some literature on the impact of use of Twitter for promotion of journal content, podcast specific data is limited. Canadian Journal of Emergency Medicine articles featured on the *Skeptics Guide to Emergency Medicine* in a "hot off the press" collaboration, showed increased abstract but not full text views when podcasts were used in comparison to social media posts alone [25]. Another retrospective study in Radiology [26] showed increased downloads and citations of articles highlighted in podcasts compared to other articles in the same issue. Neither study randomized which articles were highlighted in the podcasts and had risk of confounding as editors likely selected articles to highlight that already had potential for more downloads and citations. Matched control articles using the same topic, study design and year from International Journal of Gynecological Cancer found an increased Altmetric Attention scores(AAS) and median citations per year on podcast highlighted articles [27]. Going broader, a study using matched control articles looked at articles from five obstetrics and gynecology journal's podcasts and did not find increased AAS or citations per year when controlling for other factors [28]. Another study currently only available as an abstract looking at two oncology journals showed increased Twitter shares but no impact on citations or other measures after multivariate regression [29].

Does a Podcast Improve Dissemination?

A scoping review of podcasting for public scholarship describes how podcasting done for the purpose of dissemination of research often reaches an audience outside of the immediate community they were made for, including reaching the general public [21]. They describe podcasting as "an efficient, unifying, accessible, and multimodal means of communicating with an interested community." An individual example is the Journal of Pediatric Orthopaedics found that podcast episodes were accessed more often than the articles they covered (1236 vs. 482) supporting the idea that the podcasts can improve dissemination beyond those who are likely to read the articles [30]. While specific data may be sparse, successful podcasts reach a significant audience. For example, the American Academy of Pediatrics podcast was getting 11 K downloads per episode as a journal for a 67 K member organization [31].

Are There Risks of Podcasting for Journals or Societies?

Yes, unlike publications with established peer review processes, oversight on podcasts is variable which sets up risk. A notable example is the *JAMA Clinical Review* podcast which in 2021 had an episode on structural racism. This was promoted on Twitter with a now infamous tweet: "No physician is racist, so how can there be structural racism in healthcare?" The podcast was described as denying the existance of structral racism in medicine and the tweet and podcast were described by the AMA's chief health equity office as, "wrong, absolutely appalling and at its very core is a demonstration of structural and institutional racism." https://time.com/5956643/medical-journals-health-racism/, https://x.com/DrAlethaMaybank/status/1367501829433683968. Fallout from this tweet and episode included the editor in chief of JAMA being put on leave https://www.nytimes.com/2021/03/25/health/jama-bauchner-race-medicine.html and later stepping down as well as the AMA and JAMA demanding the deputy editor and host's resignation https://www.ama-assn.org/about/leadership/speaking-out-against-structural-racism-jama-and-across-health-care which has led to ongoing litigation. See: (*Livingston v. Am. Med. Ass'n*, No. B324638 (Cal. Ct. App. Oct. 31, 2024)) link

A reasonable goal for a journal podcast would be to get content to people who might not see the articles and to develop a sense of connection between the listeners and the journal. Podcasts are not well established as a tool to increase downloads nor citation of journal content.

Institutions

Explicit institutional affiliation is rare among top medical podcasts [8] however many podcast hosts have appointments at universities or hospital systems. The relationship of the podcasts to institutions and the apparent goals of these podcasts are variable.

Podcasts for Education Internally

Creative pedagogical applications of podcasts are all over in education at large, and are described by Cook both in the context of faculty produced content (lecture being recorded, supplementary conversation) as well as faculty mentoring students in production [3]. As early as 2006 individual educators at medical schools were pivoting from in-class to podcast based lectures with the goal of using in class time for questions and answers [32]. This is a place where we can quibble a bit about what is the definition of a podcast and if a recorded lecture is similar enough for us to combine these ideas in the same discussion. Mentored student made podcasts act to both educate the student producing the content, sometimes for internal use in the class only [33], as well as generate outward facing educational content such has been done at the University of Cincinnati [34]. Medical students producing podcasts themselves has been compared to consuming podcasts made by other students in one study with mixed results on post tests [35]. At the graduate medical education(GME) level podcasts have been used to provide content from in person conferences and used to provide more accessible content for distributed clinic sites [36, 37].

Podcasts for Medical Education and Institutional Promotion

Educational podcasts hosted in hospital or hospital systems are fairly common. Some of these seemed aimed at promotion of the institutions at large, promotion of the institutions to referring providers or for education and development of their own faculty. For example *PediacastCME* from Nationwide Children's has published on the role of hospital marketing department's support for the project [38] and Children's Hospital Philidelphia's *Primary Care Perspectives: Podcast for Pediatricians'* host is supported by the hospital for this podcast [31]. Some more pediatric examples include Children's Mercy *Pediatrics in Practice: a CME podcast*, and *The Lead in Peds* from Children's National. Additionally some hospital and university based podcasts regularly highlight research from the institution such as *That's Pediatrics* from University of Pittsburgh Medical Center's children's hospital. The impact of a podcast in promotion of a hospital or university is not well known, but it seems a well trod path with plenty of examples to point to if you are looking to garner support to start one.

Loosely Associated Podcasts with Continuing Medical Education(CME) Credits

The original Puscast (*Persiflagers Infectious Disease Puscast* 2005–2020) was a biweekly, or whichever one means every other week, podcast by Mark Crislip, which for a time provided CME through his employer Providence Healthcare. Current podcasts *Curbsiders*, and *Cribsiders* partner with Virginia Commonwealth University Health to provide CME. CME credit arrangements also exist with societies such as American College of Physicians providing CME credit for members listening to *Core IM* and *Bedside rounds*.

The percentage of people claiming CME is a tiny fraction of listeners for podcasts with CME arrangements. We have data from the institutional podcast, *PediacastCME* where only 2103 h of CME credit were claimed for 91,159 downloads [38], and *PHM from Pittsburgh* reported 1.4% of potential CME credits being obtained [39]. *Curbsiders* had 0.83% and *Cribsiders* had 0.71% of downloads associated with CME being claimed [40]. Even with limited utilization there may still be an argument to have a CME arrangement. A quality evaluation tool for online resources the rMETRIQ score includes citations and disclosures in its criteria aligning well with CME requirements [41]. The processes of making the podcasts CME eligible may add to the credibility of the podcast or the CME availability itself may increase users' perceptions of credibility.

Podcasts to Build Local Community

Podcasts are used to support developing a local community. The MacEmerg Podcast from three divisions of EM inside of MacMaster University aimed to "create a 'water cooler'–type effect" connecting members in a regionally distributed group. This group shared clinical, educational and research content relevant to regional physicians. This group highlights the high percentage of listens coming from the region of university sites as meeting this goal [42].

Commercial Educational Podcast

Commercial podcasts are a relevant slice of podcast use particularly EM:RAP which was the dominant podcast used by emergency medicine residents in a 2017 survey [43]. Commercial audio content distribution preceded the technology for podcasting. This came in the form of tapes and later cassettes in the mail with series like Practical Reviews by Educational Reviews LLC and Audiodigest; which started as edited down recordings of national conference proceedings in the 1950s [44]. By the early 1970s Audiodigest estimated reaching 150,000 physicians monthly (they claim 4 people listen to each tape) and high percentages of specialists including 41% of anesthesiologists and 36% of ophthalmologists [44]. Physical media in the mail was also the origin of the ubiquitous EM:RAP which mailed CDs. When CD-ROMS were sold for CME they also included audio lectures [45]. Downloadable MP3 files for CME were offered by other services including JournalBytes [46]. At this point there are a variety of commercial CME products some of which are audio only and podcast or at least podcast like. All this is to say physicians have long desired convenient vehicles for both ongoing learning and CME credits and podcasts are a current iteration of that.

How and Why People Are Using Podcasts for Medical Education

Why Do Listeners Use Podcasts?—Convenience, Community and Learning

A starting point is an online survey of American podcast users which describes motives for podcast listening among the general public [47]. These reasons overlap significantly with the reasons the medical education audience listens. For the general audience entertainment, escapism and information are highlighted along with podcasts being a flexible and convenient platform. They also listen to podcasts for reasons of personal/communal identification. These feelings of community and identity are important themes that also arose in interviews of emergency medicine residents who listened to medical education podcasts and found they "create a sense of connection with local peers and faculty and with the professional community at large [20]." A similar sentiment was communicated in a survey of pediatric hospitalists who felt connected to the pediatric community. Nicely described by one participant "feel less lonely in my rural community hospital; [I'm a] single pediatrician marooned among adult docs [39]." Themes from surveys and interviews of the general public, emergency medicine residents and internal medicine podcast listeners are summarized in Table 2.3. As more NotebookLM [49, 50] and other AI generated podcasts are made it will be interesting to see how acceptance of these compares to conventional human voiced podcasts.

When we podcast we are projecting the culture and values of our community to an audience who are members of the community, or maybe are considering becoming one. Interviewed EM residents talked about "learning the language" and "feeling like an insider [20]." The *Breakpoints* hosts also put this nicely in trying to share the, "water cooler conversations that all of us are already having" [12]. As such our choice of language and the culture we project are important to consider. Podcasts are also a tool for intentional culture change. They are highlighted as a way to combat racism in GME given in part to the ability to, "share perspectives that may not be available to all clinicians at their home institutions" [51].

Of course listeners see podcasts as a tool to learn. But they don't just learn in a passive continuous fashion but select content based on perceived educational needs or current cases. So while podcasts are often released on a regularly scheduled pattern their use is not always consumption in that pattern. Cribsider and Curbsider listeners claiming CME credits give the reasons for listening to an episode to be topic of interest (38%), relevance to a patient (23%), topic of less comfort (16%) all as higher reasons than just listening to the most recent episode (14%) [40]. The EM residents described an evolution for listening to a broad range of content early and later in training picking out content based on self identified gaps or recent clinical experiences [20].

Table 2.3 Motives for podcast use in a national survey [47] and themes from qualitative studies of emergency medicine residents [20] and an internal medicine podcast's listeners [48]

Convenience and entertainment—Podcasts are accessible, entertaining and fit into other daily activities like commuting, chores and household tasks. They are perceived to be efficient for learning in situations where other types of learning would not fit
Community and values—Listeners find podcasts contribute to their personal identity, affirm their values and help them feel a connection with a community in part through learning a shared language
Learning—Podcasts generally are used to keep up to date with changes in practice and literature as it is published. Specific podcasts episodes are selected to meet learning goals, and to prepare learners and educators for educational discussions

Continuing Medical Education

Post training audiences are important for many podcasts and may be along for the ride regardless of your intended primary audience. Attendings in pediatrics [39] represent about 75% of listeners to a hospital pediatrics podcast. In infectious diseases *Febrile* had 34% of its audience being faculty [1]. A large internal medicine podcast *Curbsiders* has 38% of its audience being post training representing the largest single group of their listeners [52]. The accessibility of podcasts might be particularly important for post training providers who might have less access to other educational opportunities. Physicians want to tailor their CME options to their own preferences which in some cases is an audio format when driving or on treadmill [53]. A survey of a mixed group of practicing providers in EM found podcasts to be a preferred method for continuing education [54].

Still podcasts as CME are under-investigated compared to other forms of CME; a recent scoping review of virtual CME only captured a single article on podcasting [55] and another survey of providers CME preferences did not give an option to select podcasts [56].

Integration in Graduate Medical Education

In 2020 Rodman and Trivedi described "Medical Education in 2025" as being revolutionized by organic digital education [57]. By now (2025) learners should be spending a portion of didactic time in residency using vetted materials from national experts and local instructors acting as navigators and coaches to direct them to the right materials. Publication of recommendations for how to incorporate podcasts in curriculum suggests that this is being done somewhere [58] but may not be common. In anesthesia podcast use by residents was fairly common but they were rarely assigned by the residency program [59]. Similarly in Otolaryngology podcasts use is common with only 9% reporting they heard about podcasts from faculty [60]. While residencies are not pivoting as quickly as some imagined, podcasts are being integrated, for example existing nationally produced journal podcasts for local flipped classroom sessions [61].

Largely podcast supplement curriculum for a subset of GME learners who are interested. Emergency medicine stands out as an exception where 20% of didactics can be delivered asynchronously which has led to a formal review process for the quality of potential asynchronous materials coming from free online sources in addition to post modules to meet the requirements for use [62]. Residents have limited time and only a subset will listen to a podcast recommended ad hoc or as part of a flipped classroom plan for a formal didactics. Keeping the assignment to a short episode seems to help.

Integration into Undergraduate Medical Education

It is hard to know the degree to which podcasts are used formally in undergraduate medical education. Podcasts are mentioned at times in flipped classroom literature in that students would be assigned a podcast to listen to prior to a session where active techniques were used in the classroom. Much more common are reading materials or locally recorded lectures or videos. In a flipped classroom review there is evidence for the use of video over written materials and podcasts are not mentioned [63] and another review captured a few podcast based flipped classroom interventions [64]. In one survey regarding pathology in German medical school students identified podcasts as a format they would prefer to use [65].

Independent use of podcasts by medical students is not well described. Outside of the assigned curriculum, third party resource use is common in medical students who see deficiencies in the resources provided by their medical school. Students generally hear of these from other students as opposed to faculty and in some places use of third party resources is actively discouraged [66]. Some surveys of medical students' use of online resources have not included podcasts as an option [67–69] and one survey which did include them had none of the 57 responding students using podcasts [61]. It seems likely that podcast use by students happens more often later in medical school and is directed toward content related to their intended specialty or current rotation, rather than as a supplementary resource in preclinical years. To that end 15% of *Curbsiders* listeners are students [52]. Following the lead of residents in EM 54% of applicants to EM report podcasts use outside of the formal curriculum in one abstract describing a survey of applicants [70].

How Do Listeners Use Podcast for Medical Education

While Doing Other Stuff

Surveys and interviews highlight the role of the convenience of the medium attracting learners to podcasts. Learners want to keep up with literature, fill perceived gaps and find podcasts fit into real life. They would "Rather do something than nothing [20]" and see this as a way to make the most of their time. The commute has long been perceived as wasted time. In a 1978 survey of subscribers to a cassette based review service 68% reported frequently listening in the car [71]. "I am really surprised how much time I used to waste in my car". A 1972 review describing the first 20 years of Audio Digest included details of how it was intended for use in the car as well as anecdotes such as "While jogging, I listen to Audio-Digest on a 3-pound recorder strapped to my back." and "Listen while I sit on the toilet and other such earthy times [44]."

A more contemporary interprofessional sample of emergency medicine and critical care clinicians demonstrated that often podcasts are listened to while doing other activities when listening to a sample of eight podcasts as part of the study [72]. This included driving (25.9–31.6%), doing chores (16.9–22.5%) and exercising (9.1–12.4%). With that in mind pausing and re-listening was quite variable. The use of pausing was often because of interruption but was also used intentionally for listeners to facilitate understanding. Re-listening was often because listeners felt they missed something. Taking notes was rare.

Does Listening to a Podcast While Doing Something Else Hurt Learning?

While it may seem that listening while doing other activities would lead to worse outcomes from an educational standpoint this has not borne out in two crossover studies including an randomized trial of listening seated vs driving [73] and listening seated vs aerobic exercise [74] with similar immediate and delayed post test results. Neither of these seem definitive but it is nice to not have an obvious risk here and regardless something is better than nothing, right?

How—At Increased Speed

Another commonly perceived threat to learning is the ability to listen at higher speeds. This interprofessional study had (13.9–21.3%) of podcasts listened to at above 1.5× speed or higher [72]. Similar to the 23% of participants reporting listening at increased speeds in a survey of an interprofessional group of EM and critical care medical professionals [75].

Does Listening to a Podcast at Increased Speed Hurt Learning?

The impact of playback speed has been studied more in multimedia than podcasts alone. A meta-analysis of multimedia learning studies comparing using 1× to 1.4–1.5× speed for test outcomes suggested a small negative effect on comprehension [76]. A medical education podcast specific study also showed a negative impact of increased speeds on delayed posttest scores [77]. Maybe worth thinking about for your own listening habits but not much else I can think of doing with this information on the content creation side other than making sure the intro music still sounds good at 1.5×.

Conclusion

Podcasts are largely created by individuals or groups with variable associations with institutions and journals. Journals may be using them for branding, dissemination and to engage a community around the journal while institutions are using them for education of their own faculty and trainees and promotion of the institutions. Efficacy for podcasts for any of these outcomes are not well understood. Users of podcasts largely do so for convenient self directed learning rather than formal integration of podcasts into training programs and also listen to connect, or feel connected, with local and larger communities.

References

1. Dong SW, Stead W. Impact of the febrile podcast and learning resource as an infectious diseases education platform. Open Forum Infect Dis [Internet] 2024 [cited 2025 Mar 22];11(4):ofae124. Available from: https://academic.oup.com/ofid/article/doi/10.1093/ofid/ofae124/7618907.
2. Sara Dong. Introducing Febrile, a cultured podcast [Internet]. [cited 2025 Mar 27]; Available from: https://febrilepodcast.com/episode-00-welcome-to-febrile/.
3. Cook IM. Scholarly podcasting: why, what, how? [Internet]. 1 London: Routledge; 2023 [cited 2025 Mar 22]; Available from: https://www.taylorfrancis.com/books/9781003006596.
4. Chan TM, Stehman C, Gottlieb M, Thoma B. A short history of free open access medical education. The past, present, and future. Sch [Internet] 2020 [cited 2025 Mar 22];1(2):87–100. Available from: https://www.atsjournals.org/doi/10.34197/ats-scholar.2020-0014PS.
5. Cadogan M, Thoma B, Chan TM, Lin M. Free open access meducation (FOAM): the rise of emergency medicine and critical care blogs and podcasts (2002–2013). Emerg Med J [Internet] 2014 [cited 2025 Mar 22];31(e1):e76–7. Available from: https://emj.bmj.com/lookup/doi/10.1136/emermed-2013-203502.
6. Lin M, Phipps M, Yilmaz Y, Nash CJ, Gisondi MA, Chan TM. A fork in the road for emergency medicine and critical care blogs and podcasts: cross-sectional study. JMIR Med Educ [Internet] 2022 [cited 2025 Mar 22];8(4):e39946. Available from: https://mededu.jmir.org/2022/4/e39946.
7. Oehler RL, Katzman JH, Sunny A. "Like and Subscribe": a compendium of infectious diseases audio podcasts. Open Forum Infect Dis [Internet] 2024 [cited 2025 Mar 22];11(10):ofae583. Available from: https://academic.oup.com/ofid/article/doi/10.1093/ofid/ofae583/7811604
8. Zhang E, Trad N, Corty R, Zohrob D, Trivedi S, Rodman A. How podcasts teach: A comprehensive analysis of the didactic methods of the top hundred medical podcasts. Med Teach [Internet] 2022 [cited 2025 Mar 22];44(10):1146–50. Available from: https://www.tandfonline.com/doi/full/10.1080/0142159X.2022.2071691.
9. Wilson P, Petticrew M, Booth A. After the gold rush? A systematic and critical review of general medical podcasts. J R Soc Med [Internet] 2009 [cited 2025 Mar 22];102(2):69–74. Available from: https://journals.sagepub.com/doi/10.1258/jrsm.2008.080245.
10. Clauson KA, Vidal DM. Overview of biomedical journal podcasts. Am J Health Syst Pharm [Internet] 2008 [cited 2025 Mar 22];65(22):2155–8. Available from: https://academic.oup.com/ajhp/article/65/22/2155-2158/5128149.
11. Neurology Podcast. December 11 2007 Issue [Internet]. [cited 2025 Mar 22]; Available from: https://www.neurology.org/media/podcast/december-11-2007-issue.
12. ID:IOTS podcast. IDSA difficult to treat gram negatives guidance 2024 with Breakpoints podcast [Internet]. [cited 2025 Mar 25]; Available from: https://idiotspodcasting.buzzsprout.com/1782416/episodes/16764936-104-idsa-difficult-to-treat-gram-negatives-guidance-2024-with-breakpoints-podcast.
13. Thamman R, Eshtehardi P, Narang A, Lundberg G, Khera A. Roles and impact of Journal's Social Media Editors. Circ Cardiovasc Qual Outcomes [Internet] 2021 [cited 2025 Mar 22];14(11):e007443. Available from: https://www.ahajournals.org/doi/10.1161/CIRCOUTCOMES.120.007443.

14. Cippà PE. Social Media Editor: what is it all about? Transpl Int [Internet] 2016 [cited 2025 Mar 22];29(4):390–1. Available from: https://onlinelibrary.wiley.com/doi/10.1111/tri.12762.
15. Lopez M, Chan TM, Thoma B, Arora VM, Trueger NS. The Social Media Editor at Medical Journals: responsibilities, goals, barriers, and facilitators. Acad Med [Internet] 2019 [cited 2025 Mar 22];94(5):701–7. Available from: https://journals.lww.com/00001888-201905000-00042
16. Trueger NS. Medical Journals in the age of ubiquitous social media. J Am Coll Radiol [Internet] 2018 [cited 2025 Mar 22];15(1):173–6. Available from: https://linkinghub.elsevier.com/retrieve/pii/S1546144017311924
17. Erskine N, Hendricks S. The Use of Twitter by Medical Journals: Systematic Review of the Literature. J Med Internet Res [Internet] 2021 [cited 2025 Mar 22];23(7):e26378. Available from: https://www.jmir.org/2021/7/e26378.
18. Kim D, Jung W, Jiang T, Zhu Y. An Exploratory study of Medical Journal's Twitter use: metadata, networks, and content analyses. J Med Internet Res [Internet] 2023 [cited 2025 Mar 22];25:e43521. Available from: https://www.jmir.org/2023/1/e43521.
19. Roberts LW. Academic medicine—engaging with our field through and beyond its pages. Acad Med [Internet] 2024 [cited 2025 Mar 22];99(1):1–2. Available from: https://journals.lww.com/10.1097/ACM.0000000000005506.
20. Riddell J, Robins L, Brown A, Sherbino J, Lin M, Ilgen JS. Independent and interwoven: a qualitative exploration of residents' experiences with educational podcasts. Acad Med J Assoc Am Med Coll. 2020;95(1):89–96.
21. Persohn L, Branson S. Scholarly podcasting for research dissemination: a scoping review. Sage Open [Internet] 2025 [cited 2025 Mar 22];15(1):21582440241311694. Available from: https://journals.sagepub.com/doi/10.1177/21582440241311694.
22. Hawkins CM, Hunter M, Kolenic GE, Carlos RC. Social media and peer-reviewed Medical Journal readership: a randomized prospective controlled trial. J Am Coll Radiol [Internet] 2017 [cited 2025 Mar 22];14(5):596–602. Available from: https://linkinghub.elsevier.com/retrieve/pii/S1546144016314478.
23. Fox CS, Bonaca MA, Ryan JJ, Massaro JM, Barry K, Loscalzo J. A randomized trial of social media from *Circulation*. Circulation [Internet] 2015 [cited 2025 Mar 22];131(1):28–33. Available from: https://www.ahajournals.org/doi/10.1161/CIRCULATIONAHA.114.013509
24. Fox CS, Gurary EB, Ryan J, et al. Randomized controlled trial of social media: effect of increased intensity of the intervention. J Am Heart Assoc [Internet] 2016 [cited 2025 Mar 22];5(5):e003088. Available from: https://www.ahajournals.org/doi/10.1161/JAHA.115.003088.
25. Thoma B, Murray H, Huang SYM, et al. The impact of social media promotion with infographics and podcasts on research dissemination and readership. CJEM [Internet] 2018 [cited 2025 Mar 22];20(2):300–6. Available from: https://www.cambridge.org/core/product/identifier/S1481803517003943/type/journal_article.
26. Wang M, Le T, Leswick DA. Amplifying research: the potential for podcasts to boost *Radiology* Journal article exposure. Radiology [Internet] 2024 [cited 2025 Mar 22];312(3):e233057. Available from: http://pubs.rsna.org/doi/10.1148/radiol.233057.
27. Levin G, Harrison R, Meyer R, Ramirez PT. Impact of podcasting on novel and conventional measures of academic impact. Int J Gynecol Cancer [Internet] 2023 [cited 2025 Mar 24];33(2):183–9. Available from: https://linkinghub.elsevier.com/retrieve/pii/S1048891X24009101.
28. Maxey C, Hayden J, Schneyer R, et al. The impact of obstetrics and gynecology journal podcasts on the dissemination of featured articles. Am J Obstet Gynecol MFM [Internet] 2025 [cited 2025 Mar 24];7(1):101533. Available from: https://linkinghub.elsevier.com/retrieve/pii/S2589933324002593.
29. Toussi NH, Wang YN (Richard), Jamil H, Manna M. The impact of scholarly podcasts on research distribution and uptake in oncology. JCO Oncol Pract [Internet] 2024 [cited 2025 Mar 24];20(10_suppl):423. Available from: https://ascopubs.org/doi/10.1200/OP.2024.20.10_suppl.423.

30. Paulson AE, Clement RC, Holt JB, Sanders JS, Louer CR. Orthopaedic surgery subspecialty podcast effectively disseminates peer-reviewed articles relative to traditional online publishing. J Pediatr Orthop [Internet] 2024 [cited 2025 Mar 22];44(3):e292–7. Available from: https://journals.lww.com/10.1097/BPO.0000000000002606.
31. Parga-Belinkie JJ, Cosmini M, Hill D, et al. The role of medical education podcasts in pediatrics. Pediatrics [Internet] 2023 [cited 2025 Mar 22];152(5):e2023062911. Available from: https://publications.aap.org/pediatrics/article/152/5/e2023062911/194491/The-Role-of-Medical-Education-Podcasts-in.
32. Podcast lectures for uni students [Internet]. BBC News. 2006 [cited 2025 Feb 5]; Available from: http://news.bbc.co.uk/2/hi/uk_news/england/west_yorkshire/5013194.stm.
33. Nie M, Cashmore A, Cane C. The educational value of student generated podcasts [Internet]. In: ALT-C 2008 Research Proceedings. Leeds UK: Available from: https://repository.alt.ac.uk/438/1/ALT_C_2008_rp_mingn_cashmorea_canec.pdf.
34. Milligan KJ, Daulton RS, St Clair ZT, Epperson MV, Holloway RM, Schlaudecker JD. Creation of a Student-Run Medical Education Podcast: Tutorial. JMIR Med Educ [Internet] 2021 [cited 2025 Mar 22];7(3):e29157. Available from: https://mededu.jmir.org/2021/3/e29157.
35. Laupichler MC, Aster A, Soyubey L, et al. Influence of active production versus passive consumption of podcasts on medical students' learning outcomes. Clin Teach [Internet] 2025 [cited 2025 Mar 22];22(1):e70029. Available from: https://asmepublications.onlinelibrary.wiley.com/doi/10.1111/tct.70029.
36. Shekarchi A, Gordon B, Liu J. Using podcasts in place of clinic talks for graduate medical education at a multi-site residency program. Pediatrics [Internet] 2018 [cited 2025 Mar 22];142(1_MeetingAbstract):620. Available from: https://publications.aap.org/pediatrics/article/142/1_MeetingAbstract/620/2816/Using-Podcasts-in-Place-of-Clinic-Talks-for.
37. Childers RE, Dattalo M, Christmas C. Podcast pearls in residency training. Ann Intern Med [Internet] 2014 [cited 2025 Mar 31];160(1):70–1. Available from: https://www.acpjournals.org/doi/10.7326/L14-5000-2.
38. Patrick MD, Stukus DR, Nuss KE. Using podcasts to deliver pediatric educational content: development and reach of PediaCast CME. Digit Health [Internet] 2019 [cited 2025 Mar 22];5:2055207619834842. Available from: https://journals.sagepub.com/doi/10.1177/2055207619834842.
39. Tarchichi TR, Szymusiak J. Attending physician's attitudes toward podcasting as a source of medical education: an exploratory study. J Contin Educ Health Prof [Internet] 2020 [cited 2025 Mar 22];40(2):141–4. Available from: https://journals.lww.com/10.1097/CEH.0000000000000291.
40. Kelly JM, Perseghin A, Dow A, et al. Continuing education evaluations of an internal medicine and a pediatric podcast. J Contin Educ Health Prof [Internet] 2023 [cited 2025 Mar 24];43(4):283–6. Available from: https://journals.lww.com/10.1097/CEH.0000000000000501.
41. Colmers-Gray IN, Krishnan K, Chan TM, et al. The revised METRIQ score: a quality evaluation tool for online educational resources. AEM Educ Train [Internet] 2019 [cited 2025 Mar 22];3(4):387–92. Available from: https://onlinelibrary.wiley.com/doi/10.1002/aet2.10376.
42. Dong JK, Khalid M, Murdock M, et al. MacEmerg Podcast: a novel initiative to connect a distributed community of practice. AEM Educ Train [Internet] 2021 [cited 2025 Mar 22];5(3):e10550. Available from: https://onlinelibrary.wiley.com/doi/10.1002/aet2.10550.
43. Riddell J, Swaminathan A, Lee M, Mohamed A, Rogers R, Rezaie S. A survey of emergency medicine residents' use of educational podcasts. West J Emerg Med [Internet] 2017 [cited 2025 Mar 22];18(2):229–34. Available from: http://escholarship.org/uc/item/4fg852z1.
44. Oakley CL. The first twenty years of audio-digest. Calif Med. 1972;116(6):81–8.
45. Mullich J, Groveman H. Virtual CME: better than being there. Phys Sportsmed [Internet] 1996 [cited 2025 Mar 25];24(sup1):25–30. Available from: https://www.tandfonline.com/doi/full/10.1080/00913847.1996.11948072.
46. Wheeler D. CME credit for pathology journal review. Adv Anat Pathol. 2006;13(3):139–40.

47. Chan-Olmsted S, Wang R. Understanding podcast users: Consumption motives and behaviors. New Media Soc [Internet] 2022 [cited 2025 Mar 22];24(3):684–704. Available from: https://journals.sagepub.com/doi/10.1177/1461444820963776.
48. Malecki SL, Quinn KL, Zilbert N, et al. Understanding the use and perceived impact of a medical podcast: qualitative study. JMIR Med Educ [Internet] 2019 [cited 2025 Nov 13];5(2):e12901. Available from: http://mededu.jmir.org/2019/2/e12901/.
49. Tejani AS, Khosravi B, Savage CH, Moy L, Kahn CE, Yi PH. AI-generated podcast summaries of *Radiology* articles: analysis of content and quality. Radiology [Internet] 2025 [cited 2025 Mar 24];314(3):e243270. Available from: http://pubs.rsna.org/doi/10.1148/radiol.243270.
50. Dihan QA, Nihalani BR, Tooley AA, Elhusseiny AM. Eyes on Google's NotebookLM: using generative AI to create ophthalmology podcasts with a single click. Eye [Internet] 2025 [cited 2025 Mar 24];39(2):215–6. Available from: https://www.nature.com/articles/s41433-024-03481-8.
51. Kamal S, Trivedi SP, Essien UR, Nematollahi S. Podcasting: a medium for amplifying racial justice discourse, reflection, and representation within graduate medical education. J Grad Med Educ [Internet] 2021 [cited 2025 Mar 29];13(1):29–32. Available from: https://meridian.allenpress.com/jgme/article/13/1/29/451598/Podcasting-A-Medium-for-Amplifying-Racial-Justice.
52. Berk J, Trivedi SP, Watto M, Williams P, Centor R. Medical education podcasts: where we are and questions unanswered. J Gen Intern Med [Internet] 2020 [cited 2025 Mar 22];35(7):2176–8. Available from: http://link.springer.com/10.1007/s11606-019-05606-2.
53. Young KJ, Kim JJ, Yeung G, Sit C, Tobe SW. Physician Preferences for Accredited Online Continuing Medical Education. J Contin Educ Health Prof [Internet] 2011 [cited 2025 Mar 30];31(4):241–6. Available from: https://journals.lww.com/00005141-201131040-00004.
54. Kalnow A, Beck-Esmay J, Riddell J, et al. Continuing medical education delivery preferences among physicians and advanced practice providers in emergency medicine. Cureus [Internet] 2021 [cited 2025 Mar 22]; Available from: https://www.cureus.com/articles/79501-continuing-medical-education-delivery-preferences-among-physicians-and-advanced-practice-providers-in-emergency-medicine.
55. Cheng C, Papadakos J, Umakanthan B, et al. On the advantages and disadvantages of virtual continuing medical education: a scoping review. Can Med Educ J. 2023;14(3):41–74.
56. O'Brien Pott M, Blanshan AS, Huneke KM, Baasch Thomas BL, Cook DA. What influences choice of continuing medical education modalities and providers? A National Survey of U.S. Physicians, Nurse Practitioners, and Physician Assistants. Acad Med [Internet] 2021 [cited 2025 Mar 24];96(1):93–100. Available from: https://journals.lww.com/10.1097/ACM.0000000000003758.
57. Rodman A, Trivedi S. Podcasting: a roadmap to the future of medical education. Semin Nephrol [Internet] 2020 [cited 2025 Mar 22];40(3):279–83. Available from: https://linkinghub.elsevier.com/retrieve/pii/S0270929520300474.
58. Chaiklin C, Onyango J, Heublein M, Gielissen K, Kryzhanovskaya I (Era). Twelve tips for integrating podcasts into medical education curricula. Med Teach [Internet] 2024 [cited 2025 Mar 22];46(5):621–5. Available from: https://www.tandfonline.com/doi/full/10.1080/0142159X.2023.2280118.
59. Anesthesia Learning in the Digital Age: Are Program Directors and Residents on the Same Page? J Educ Perioper Med [Internet] 2020 [cited 2025 Mar 22];22(2). Available from: https://www.seahq.org/assets/docs/volxxii_issue2_wolpaw.pdf.
60. Vanstrum EB, Badash I, Wu FM, et al. The role of educational podcast use among otolaryngology residents. Ann Otol Rhinol Laryngol [Internet] 2022 [cited 2025 Mar 24];131(12):1353–7. Available from: http://journals.sagepub.com/doi/10.1177/00034894211072996.
61. Ratliff JB, Nascimento FA, Tornes L, et al. Curriculum innovations: a podcast-based neurologic emergency flipped classroom curriculum for neurology residents. Neurol Educ [Internet] 2023

[cited 2025 Mar 22];2(3):e200081. Available from: https://www.neurology.org/doi/10.1212/NE9.0000000000200081.
62. Lin M, Joshi N, Grock A, et al. Approved instructional resources series: a national initiative to identify quality emergency medicine blog and podcast content for resident education. J Grad Med Educ [Internet] 2016 [cited 2025 Mar 22];8(2):219–25. Available from: https://meridian.allenpress.com/jgme/article/8/2/219/34504/Approved-Instructional-Resources-Series-A-National.
63. Oudbier J, Spaai G, Timmermans K, Boerboom T. Enhancing the effectiveness of flipped classroom in health science education: a state-of-the-art review. BMC Med Educ [Internet] 2022 [cited 2025 Mar 25];22(1):34. Available from: https://bmcmededuc.biomedcentral.com/articles/10.1186/s12909-021-03052-5.
64. Ramnanan C, Pound L. Advances in medical education and practice: student perceptions of the flipped classroom. Adv Med Educ Pract [Internet] 2017 [cited 2025 Mar 25];Volume 8:63–73. Available from: https://www.dovepress.com/advances-in-medical-education-and-practice-student-perceptions-of-the%2D%2Dpeer-reviewed-article-AMEP.
65. Herrmann FEM, Lenski M, Steffen J, et al. A survey study on student preferences regarding pathology teaching in Germany: a call for curricular modernization. BMC Med Educ [Internet] 2015 [cited 2025 Mar 31];15(1):94. Available from: https://bmcmededuc.biomedcentral.com/articles/10.1186/s12909-015-0381-7.
66. Lawrence ECN, Dine CJ, Kogan JR. Preclerkship medical students' use of third-party learning resources. JAMA Netw Open [Internet] 2023 [cited 2025 Mar 27];6(12):e2345971. Available from: https://jamanetwork.com/journals/jamanetworkopen/fullarticle/2812522.
67. Judd T, Elliott K. Selection and use of online learning resources by first-year medical students: cross-sectional study. JMIR Med Educ [Internet] 2017 [cited 2025 Mar 27];3(2):e17. Available from: http://mededu.jmir.org/2017/2/e17/.
68. Wynter L, Burgess A, Kalman E, Heron JE, Bleasel J. Medical students: what educational resources are they using? BMC Med Educ [Internet] 2019 [cited 2025 Mar 27];19(1):36. Available from: https://bmcmededuc.biomedcentral.com/articles/10.1186/s12909-019-1462-9.
69. Scott K, Morris A, Marais B. Medical student use of digital learning resources. Clin Teach [Internet] 2018 [cited 2025 Mar 27];15(1):29–33. Available from: https://onlinelibrary.wiley.com/doi/10.1111/tct.12630.
70. Lee, T, Rosen, C. Curricular and co-curricular social media-based learning during medical school. West J Emerg Med Integrating Emerg Care Popul Health [Internet] 2017;(18(5.1)). Available from: https://escholarship.org/uc/item/6vq820fh.
71. Scott LK, Brascho DJ, Brown S. An evaluation of the effectiveness of audio cassettes for CME. Med Educ [Internet] 1978 [cited 2025 Mar 22];12(6):427–30. Available from: https://onlinelibrary.wiley.com/doi/10.1111/j.1365-2923.1978.tb01422.x.
72. Roland D, Thoma B, Tagg A, Woods J, Chan TM, Riddell J. What are the real-world podcast-listening habits of medical professionals? Cureus [Internet] 2021 [cited 2025 Mar 22]; Available from: https://www.cureus.com/articles/62158-what-are-the-real-world-podcast-listening-habits-of-medical-professionals.
73. Gottlieb M, Riddell J, Cooney R, King A, Fung C-C, Sherbino J. Maximizing the morning commute: a randomized trial assessing the effect of driving on podcast knowledge acquisition and retention. Ann Emerg Med [Internet] 2021 [cited 2025 Mar 22];78(3):416–24. Available from: https://linkinghub.elsevier.com/retrieve/pii/S0196064421001621.
74. Gottlieb M, Cooney R, Haas MRC, King A, Fung C-C, Riddell J. A randomized trial assessing the effect of exercise on residents' podcast knowledge acquisition and retention. Acad Med [Internet] 2024 [cited 2025 Mar 22];99(5):575–81. Available from: https://journals.lww.com/10.1097/ACM.0000000000005592.
75. Thoma B, Goerzen S, Horeczko T, et al. An international, interprofessional investigation of the self-reported podcast listening habits of emergency clinicians: a METRIQ Study. CJEM

[Internet] 2020 [cited 2025 Mar 22];22(1):112–7. Available from: https://www.cambridge.org/core/product/identifier/S1481803519004275/type/journal_article.

76. Cheng L, Pastore R, Ritzhaupt AD. Examining the accelerated playback hypothesis of time-compression in multimedia learning environments: a meta-analysis study. J Educ Comput Res [Internet] 2022 [cited 2025 Mar 22];60(3):579–98. Available from: https://journals.sagepub.com/doi/10.1177/07356331211043535.
77. Krokar L, Atkinson AG, Nguyen DT, Willis RE. The effect of listening speed on comprehension: are you sacrificing comprehension by speeding up? Glob Surg Educ – J Assoc Surg Educ [Internet] 2023 [cited 2025 Mar 22];3(1):13. Available from: https://link.springer.com/10.1007/s44186-023-00213-6.

Chapter 3
Making Medical Education Podcasts for Patients

Kishore Vellody

Medical Education Podcasts for Patients

In their over two decades of existence, podcasts have grown exponentially in their popularity and into our daily lives. It is rare to find someone with a smartphone who doesn't regularly listen to at least one podcast. In the field of medical education, they play a vital role in disseminating information to trainees and healthcare professionals. The past decade has seen a rapid increase in use and uptake of podcasts for medical students, residents, attendings and other clinicians [1, 2]. However, the impact of medical podcasts designed specifically for the general population remains largely unexplored. Clinical providers interested in podcasting should note that there is currently no data showing a quantifiable effect on patient health and well-being from podcasts designed to deliver medical information. Despite the lack of known impact, many hospital systems have incorporated patient facing podcasts into their media outputs.

The central question remains: can podcasts truly empower patients and families to better understand and manage medical conditions? Is there value for a patient or family to listen to a podcast that further discusses their diagnosed medical conditions? Does access to more medical information via a podcast allow a patient to more fully understand their medical conditions? Could having added information potentially impact medical outcomes by encouraging patients and family to ask questions and engage in improved preventative care during clinic visits? While

K. Vellody (✉)
University of Pittsburgh School of Medicine, Pittsburgh, PA, USA

UPMC Children's Hospital of Pittsburgh – Paul C. Gaffney Division of Pediatric Hospital Medicine, Pittsburgh, PA, USA

Down Syndrome Center of Western Pennsylvania, Pittsburgh, PA, USA
e-mail: vellodyk@upmc.edu

J. Parga-Belinkie et al. (eds.), *Podcasting for Medical Professionals*,
https://doi.org/10.1007/978-3-032-16480-3_3

evidence-based answers to these questions remain elusive, common sense suggests that providing evidence-based medical content is a form of public health messaging and should, therefore, improve patient outcomes. With regards to an individual patient receiving optimal care, their ability to more thoroughly understand their conditions and treatment options could clearly be a tremendous advantage in their care—both how they receive it and their trust in the medical system.

A Case Study: Podcasting for Families of Children with Down Syndrome

Beyond the Clinical Visit: Empowering Families Through Podcasting

Children with complex healthcare needs require improved systems to ensure optimal health care [3]. Down syndrome is the most common genetic condition resulting in intellectual disability with approximately 1 in every 775 liveborn babies having Down syndrome [4]. There are an estimated 220,000 individuals with Down syndrome living in the United States today, many of whom have complex healthcare needs [5]. There are 200–300 genes found on chromosome 21, and the added gene products translate to a variety of potential medical conditions throughout the lifespan of someone with Down syndrome. Individuals with Down syndrome may face various medical conditions, including congenital heart disease, hematologic/oncologic disorders, hypothyroidism, hearing and vision deficits, and overall developmental delays in gross motor, fine motor, and expressive speech production. The American Academy of Pediatrics first published health supervision recommendations for children with Down syndrome in 1999, most recently revised in 2022 [6]. Similarly, the first evidence-based adult healthcare guideline for Down syndrome was published in 2020 [7]. These comprehensive recommendations cover many of the major medical, developmental, and behavioral issues that can arise over the lifetime in someone with Down syndrome. However, in this modern era of healthcare delivery, there is often less time available during individual outpatient clinic visits than ever before. Healthcare professionals often feel rushed during the shorter visits leading to missed opportunities for patient education, incomplete assessments, and increased anxiety for families. It is no surprise that patient satisfaction with clinician visits also suffers in this model [8]. In caring for a patient with Down syndrome who may also have added medical complexities, the additional guideline-based recommendations may be overwhelming to complete with the time constraints present. Despite medical providers reporting adequate knowledge of the guideline recommendations, their patients are rarely fully up to date with those recommendations, in part due to these time restrictions [9–11]. Fifty percent of guardians of a loved one with Down syndrome are unaware of the available medical guidelines [12]. Therefore, patients and families turn to general internet search engines for information and often will find inaccurate and non-evidence based information. Even if they find accurate information, it can consist of overly complex articles filled with difficult-to-understand medical terminology and jargon.

Recognizing the need for improved healthcare for people with Down syndrome, the Down Syndrome Center of Western Pennsylvania (DSC) was founded by parents, family members, and people with Down syndrome in the western Pennsylvania region. These pioneering families recognized, even long before there was published healthcare guidance, that their family members with Down syndrome needed specialized healthcare. They knew that even the busiest of pediatric health care professionals would, based on statistical average, see at most three to four patients with Down syndrome per year. The combination of the low volume of patients with Down syndrome seen, and the limited time with which to see them, meant innovation was necessary for optimal healthcare of their loved ones with Down syndrome. These local families (of what would become known as the Down Syndrome Association of Pittsburgh) did the initial grassroots fundraising that resulted in the creation of the DSC at the Children's Hospital of Pittsburgh which first began seeing patients in September 1989. As a result, children and adults with Down syndrome in our region can receive specific and specialized Down syndrome related care without the patients, families, or providers feeling the time restrictions that would otherwise be present. With this dedicated team and the philanthropic support, the DSC provides tailored care, allowing more time for patient interactions than typical outpatient settings.

Medical professionals often wish they had more time with patients to address healthcare issues, but families of children with Down syndrome needed more than just extended exam room visits. Even with the additional time availability afforded the DSC through the philanthropy, questions still arose that could not be completely answered during a visit. Parents might wonder about the best toilet training methods for children with Down syndrome, how to transition their child from preschool to kindergarten, or what college programs are available for young adults. These types of parenting quandaries often arise in the middle of the night, when anxiety is high but the issue is not urgent enough to warrant calling the doctor. These topics also have many potential individualized responses and don't lend themselves to quick, universal answers. Given their popularity and ease of access, a podcast seemed to be the most efficient and thorough way to address these common questions in an easily distributed format. However, a search for "Down syndrome" in a podcast index in the year 2013 resulted in 2 podcasts, and neither covered medically related information. Therefore, the DSC became determined to fill that void and created a podcast to provide families with essential information families could access outside of the clinic walls.

The first step was to secure institutional support from within the academic division. Next, funding was secured to obtain the necessary recording equipment, including a laptop and a microphone. The patients and families of the DSC were polled for the most important topics that they would like the podcasts to cover. Expert guests were identified and requested to join the podcast to share their knowledge. At first, the podcast was recorded in-person with an informal question and answer format. Over time, online recording became the preferred format (more below). Libsyn (https://www.libysn.com) was chosen as the online podcast host site. In February 2013, the first episode of the Down Syndrome Center Podcast was released.

The initial aim was for the podcast to reach the local families cared for at the DSC with easily understood information provided without overly complex medical terminology resulting in "jargon oblivion." [13] However, it quickly gained a national and international audience. Twelve years since the first episode was released, nearly 200 podcasts have been released and downloaded in over 100 countries, with over 260,000 total downloads. About 90% of the downloads are from outside of the podcast's home state of Pennsylvania, and 25% of the downloads are from outside of the United States. Each podcast concludes with a request for the listeners to send in questions that they would like addressed on a future podcast. Listeners from all over the globe have reached out with questions to address on the podcast. This has been especially powerful since specialized Down Syndrome Centers are rare in most parts of the world. Even within the US, there are only an estimated 76 Down Syndrome Centers nationwide with 15 states without any Down Syndrome Center within their borders. Between 35% and 44% of individuals with Down syndrome must travel over 2 hours to reach their nearest Down Syndrome Center [14, 15]. Both nationally and internationally, there is a need for accurate and up-to-date information on Down syndrome that may not be able to be obtained in an in-person clinic visit. The DSC Podcast was not geographically constrained and has been able provide expert answers to questions that otherwise would not have been possible.

Adapting Recordings in a Digital Ecosystem

Initially, the podcast required guests to be local for in-person recordings, scheduled at a mutually convenient time and place. This approach worked well until the COVID-19 pandemic. The pandemic significantly altered podcasting, making in-person recordings impossible and prompting most podcasters to switch to online alternatives. Within days of pandemic restrictions being implemented, the Down Syndrome Center Podcast transitioned to Zoom for recordings. While initially presenting technical hurdles, this shift unexpectedly broadened the podcast's reach, allowing us to invite national and international experts to share their knowledge on listener-requested topics. As more experts were able to join remotely as guests on the podcasts, the episode topics broadened considerably. Podcasts on the latest information in Alzheimer dementia, Down Syndrome Regression Disorder, sleep apnea, obesity management, and autoimmunity treatments have served to bring an entire community together with the latest medical information. Many of these topics included guests who were actively recruiting patients with Down syndrome into their studies, and this information was helpful for them in letting the community know about these studies.

Some of the most impactful podcasts have been from an advocacy perspective. There are several Down syndrome focused national advocacy organizations who engage in critical work around improving the lives of people with Down syndrome across the country. The DSC podcast was able to have representatives from the National Down Syndrome Congress, National Down Syndrome Society, Global Down Syndrome Foundation, Down Syndrome Affiliates in Action, Jack's Basket, and the Down Syndrome Diagnosis Network come onto the podcast and discuss their work. These national leaders were able to discuss their work and garner support for important congressional bills. They were also able to discuss their organizations' available resources and share information on upcoming community events. Many of these experts also discussed their work in educational advocacy and classroom inclusion. They provided best practices on how school administrators and teachers could educate students with Down syndrome in the least restrictive environment.

From the outset, the Down Syndrome Center Podcast has not been academic in a traditional sense. To this day, the intended audience continues to be patients and family members of people with Down syndrome. All guests are instructed to share information using patient and family-centered language and to communicate difficult concepts as if they are speaking to a non-medical audience. While the podcast does have many regular listeners who are medical professionals, the topics covered are those of interest to patients and families. However, an unanticipated benefit of hosting the podcast was the host's emergence as a nationally recognized expert in the field. The host has been invited to serve on several national boards and has been a highly sought speaker for a variety of national and international conferences. In times where academic promotion is predicated on national recognition, national letters of support for promotion are critical. Hosting a nationally recognized podcast, even one for patients and families, can significantly contribute to an academic promotion portfolio, as demonstrated by the DSC Podcast.

Lessons Learned: Starting a Parent Facing Podcast

The Down Syndrome Center Podcast aims to inspire medical professionals to create podcasts for patients and their families. Podcasting for the public can serve several functions:

- **Raising awareness** for lesser-known medical conditions
- **Providing accessible, in-depth content** to be provided outside of the healthcare system
- **Translating complicated medical terminology** into conversational language
- **Fostering community** among listeners

When considering a medical education podcasts for patients, medical professionals must first identify their "why." A clear vision for the podcast's impact will make it mission-driven and a powerful vehicle for advocacy. Knowing your audience will enable the creation of the most impactful podcast episodes, open avenues for growth, and build a dedicated listenership invested in the content and its reach.

Conclusion

Podcasts have become a well-recognized component of medical education since they first began over two decades ago. While their contribution to the academic education landscape is now known, their potential impact in patient and family clinical education remains largely unstudied. The Down Syndrome Center Podcast has shown how a medical-themed podcast can reach a global community of people with crucial information for the care of their loved ones. It has also demonstrated that this endeavor can also result in academic advancement for a clinician who is hosting the podcast as well. More data is needed to quantify the effects, but podcasts are a clear tool to reach patients and families with information on medical, developmental, behavioral, advocacy, and educational efforts. Other healthcare providers should strongly consider employing the use of podcasts to disseminate information to their patients and families.

References

1. Kelly JM, Perseghin A, Dow AW, Trivedi SP, Rodman A, Berk J. Learning through listening: a scoping review of podcast use in medical education. Acad Med. 2022;97(7):1079–85. https://doi.org/10.1097/ACM.0000000000004565. Epub 2022 Jun 23. PMID: 34935729; PMCID: PMC11002568.
2. Riddell J, Robins L, Brown A, Sherbino J, Lin M, Ilgen JS. Independent and interwoven: a qualitative exploration of residents' experiences with educational podcasts. Acad Med. 2020;95:89–96.
3. Elias ER, Murphy NA, Council on Children with Disabilities. Home care of children and youth with complex health care needs and technology dependencies. Pediatrics. 2012;129(5):996–1005. https://doi.org/10.1542/peds.2012-0606. Epub 2012 Apr 30.
4. de Graaf G, Buckley F, Skotko BG. Estimates of the live births, natural losses, and elective terminations with Down syndrome in the United States. Am J Med Genet A. 2015;167A(4):756–67. https://doi.org/10.1002/ajmg.a.37001.
5. de Graaf G, Buckley F, Dever J, Skotko BG. Estimation of live birth and population prevalence of Down syndrome in nine U.S. states. Am J Med Genet A. 2017;173(10):2710–9. https://doi.org/10.1002/ajmg.a.38402. Epub 2017 Aug 16.
6. Bull MJ, Trotter T, Santoro SL, Christensen C, Grout RW, Council on Genetics, Burke LW, Berry SA, Geleske TA, Holm I, Hopkin RJ, Introne WJ, Lyons MJ, Monteil DC, Scheuerle A, Stoler JM, Vergano SA, Chen E, Hamid R, Downs SM, Grout RW, Cunniff C, Parisi MA, Ralston SJ, Scott JA, Shapira SK, Spire P. Health supervision for children and adolescents with down syndrome. Pediatrics. 2022;149(5):e2022057010. https://doi.org/10.1542/peds.2022-057010.

7. Tsou AY, Bulova P, Capone G, Chicoine B, Gelaro B, Harville TO, Martin BA, McGuire DE, McKelvey KD, Peterson M, Tyler C, Wells M, Whitten MS, Global Down Syndrome Foundation Medical Care Guidelines for Adults with Down Syndrome Workgroup. Medical care of adults with down syndrome: a clinical guideline. JAMA. 2020;324(15):1543–56. https://doi.org/10.1001/jama.2020.17024.
8. Geraghty EM, Franks P, Kravitz RL. Primary care visit length, quality, and satisfaction for standardized patients with depression. J Gen Intern Med. 2007;22(12):1641–7. https://doi.org/10.1007/s11606-007-0371-5. Epub 2007 Oct 6. PMID: 17922171; PMCID: PMC2219826.
9. Santoro SL, Yin H, Hopkin RJ. Adherence to symptom-based care guidelines for down syndrome. Clin Pediatr (Phila). 2017;56(2):150–6. https://doi.org/10.1177/0009922816652416. Epub 2016 Jul 19.
10. Wood JC, Gochyyev P, Santoro SL. Adherence to adult clinical practice guidelines for Down syndrome. Am J Med Genet A. 2025;197(1):e63850. https://doi.org/10.1002/ajmg.a.63850. Epub 2024 Aug 29.
11. Santoro SL, Martin LJ, Pleatman SI, Hopkin RJ. Stakeholder buy-in and physician education improve adherence to guidelines for down syndrome. J Pediatr. 2016;171:262–8.e1-2. https://doi.org/10.1016/j.jpeds.2015.12.026. Epub 2016 Jan 29.
12. Eaves L, Ho H, Laird B, Dickson S. Raising a child with down syndrome: parents' evaluations of health information and support. Downs Syndr Res Pract. 1996;4(2):65–9. https://doi.org/10.3104/reports.64.
13. Pitt MB, Hendrickson MA. Eradicating Jargon-Oblivion-A proposed classification system of medical Jargon. J Gen Intern Med. 2020;35(6):1861–4. https://doi.org/10.1007/s11606-019-05526-1. Epub 2019 Nov 11. PMID: 31713041; PMCID: PMC7280401.
14. Joslyn N, Berger H, Skotko BG. Geospatial analyses of accessibility to down syndrome specialty care. J Pediatr. 2020;218:146–150.e1. https://doi.org/10.1016/j.jpeds.2019.10.058.
15. Jensen K, Llamas P, Howard J, Berger H, Skotko B. Specialty care oases: utilizing geographic information systems to evaluate specialty care access for individuals with down syndrome. Am J Med Genet A. 2024:e63977. https://doi.org/10.1002/ajmg.a.63977. Epub ahead of print.

Chapter 4
Podcast Structure

Tony Tarchichi

Introduction

Podcasts vary in their length, the composition of their hosts, use of guests and their audience or intended reach. Medical podcasts cater to a variety of different audiences and must alter their structure to suit the needs of their listenership.

Episode Duration

The length of an educational podcast has been discussed in the literature and evolved over time as medical podcasting has become more popular. The early literature supported a podcast for education should be no longer than a song, approximately 4 min [1]. That was based mostly on expert opinion.

These early studies in podcasting focused on high school and then undergraduate students . As the audience changed to include an older demographic, the time lengthened. A new benchmark of 15 min or less became a good length for an educational podcast. Often cited was the data on adult learning theory that past 20 min lectures become less effective and the adult learner would be unable to absorb the information [2]. A 2013 survey study of Canadian Anesthesia residents felt 5 to 15 min was the perfect length of time for an educational podcast [3].

T. Tarchichi (✉)
Department of Pediatrics, University of Pittsburgh School of Medicine, Pittsburgh, PA, USA

UPMC Children's Hospital of Pittsburgh, Paul C. Gaffney Division of Pediatric Hospital Medicine, Pittsburgh, PA, USA
e-mail: tarchichitr@upmc.edu

J. Parga-Belinkie et al. (eds.), *Podcasting for Medical Professionals*,
https://doi.org/10.1007/978-3-032-16480-3_4

More recent data has supported a longer length to promote medical education. PHM from Pittsburgh is a longer length medical education podcast that has an average episode length of 60 min. A survey study from 2020 showed 77% of its listeners felt the podcast length was just right [4]. This tell us that while there is data to guide us, there isn't a one size fits all answer to podcast length. Additionally, over time listeners have been more accepting of longer podcast episodes. The details of the intended audience, reason for the podcast and format must all be taken into consideration when thinking about how long your episodes should run.

For the medical educator, ask why the learners are listening to your podcast. Is this part of a curriculum or class they are taking? Is this supplementing learning material they are required to learn for a program or course? Then we recommend 15 to 20 min or less for your podcast episode length. Tell them what they need to know, you can try to be entertaining, but brevity is key here. If the podcast you are making is optional for learners to learn a subject in more detail, then you can have longer episodes being mindful of keeping your listener attentive and interested.

Let's again use the PHM from Pittsburgh podcast as a case study. It was initially created for pediatric hospitalists to better take care of hospitalized children and remains the only podcast created for that specific sub-specialty. The listeners are hearing topics relevant to their daily work with detailed evidence-based medicine reviews and expert commentary. This follows with adult learning theories six cardinal learning related factors: the need to know, the learner's self-concept, the role of learner's experiences, readiness to learn, orientation to learning and motivation [2]. As such the 60 min run times are tolerated and enjoyed by this very targeted audience.

Structure

When discussing the structure of a podcast, there are three major categories to consider: monologue, dialogue, and panel discussions.

A monologue is one person talking the entire time. Dialogue could be a conversations between two regular hosts or refer to a host and a guest format, where the guest is often an expert in the medical topic being discussed. Lastly, panel discussion podcasts are a dynamic and conversational style of podcast where a group of individuals—usually three or more—engage in a guided discussion around a central theme or topic.

Monologue podcasts are rarer now due to the reasons listed above. Now, with the ability of artificial intelligence (AI) to create podcasts, personalized monologue podcasts are being created for rapid review of material for an exam. AI allows you to take your notes for an exam and create a podcast reviewing the material. While these are not being disseminated widely, we feel this usage deserves mention given it can be an effective learning tool.

Early literature compared monologue and dialogue and clearly showed learners prefer **dialogue podcasts** [5]. In the early days of podcasting (from 2000 to 2010), medical educators were using monologue formats by recording lectures and

Table 4.1 Comparison of podcast structure

Format	Strengths in medical education	Potential challenges
Monologue	Clear, concise, good for revision	Dry or less engaging
Dialogue	Relatable, allows for storytelling	May lack depth if not well-structured
Panel discussion	Diverse perspectives, dynamic conversation	Risk of going off-topic or overwhelming the listener

releasing them an audio tracks. These early forays into podcasting were not popular and did not last. Learners overall prefer podcasts to be approachable and conversational. The most popular dialogue formats are when the host is at the training level of the audience, and the guest is an expert in the area they are discussing [5]. This is typically a two person show, regular host or rotation of hosts but one at a time with one expert guest. This format allows for a deeper dive into a topic and a more personal feel. It facilitates storytelling due to the smaller group, and stories tend to resonate with listeners and help them absorb medical information. The potential limitations to this type of structure are it requires significant preparation in the topic of interest by the host (scripting questions, understanding flow), and the expert must be both knowledgeable and engaging, which can be difficult to find.

Panel discussions will have three or more voices which can bring a range of opinions and experiences and more of a diversity of views and voices. This format allows for more free flowing conversation. A potential limitation is the conversation veering from the intended learning topic, and an inability to provide depth for the listener.

Please see Table 4.1 for a summary of all three podcast structures.

Content and Audience

One of the first recommendations when deciding to create a podcast for medical education is to decide on its intended audience. Be as specific as possible. The audience's motivation for listening to your podcast will guide you in what material you cover and how you present it. For example, a podcast intended for parents of a child with Down syndrome discussing the atrio-ventricular cardiac anomalies with this condition will have a different level of detail than if that same podcast episode was intended for pediatric cardiologists. See Table 4.2 below for more details. It discusses in detail differing groups may expect different material presented on the same condition, depending on their motivation and needs.

Questions to Ask About Your Audience

1. What level of training are they: students, residents, fellows, attending physicians, nurses, advanced practice providers, physicians' assistants, respiratory therapists, physical therapists, dentists, etc.?

Table 4.2 Audience type and motivation for listening to medical education podcast

Audience type	Motivation	Presentation style
Parent or patient	Learn more about their condition and/or family members' condition and how to best manage it/what to expect	Giving background and understanding Focus discussion on prognosis, making the diagnosis, treatment and anything concerning Give practical information that can be acted upon such as where a person should go if they are concerned
Learner in a course/class	Improve their knowledge and understanding Get a better grade or pass an important exam Required part of their curriculum	Give more detail on the pathogenesis or background science of the topic Can give examples of how it can be tested in an exam If required—consider at shorter length of 15 to 20 min
Health care professional	Improve their knowledge and understanding of a condition to take care of their patients better	Give significant details and an explanation Go over background data and research If there are guidelines from a governing body, review them Give clinical examples and allow for storytelling, Can consider a longer format of up to 60 min

   (a) Recognize that the more specialized the audience you choose for your podcast (i.e. pediatric cardiology attendings) the more likely you are to have those not at that level listening (i.e. medical students, residents and nurses). The same is not true in reverse order. A podcast for a medical student will likely have proportionately less residents and attending physicians listening.

2. Are they obligated to listen to (Like part of a class or course they must take) or is it optional (something they are choosing to listen to on their own time)?

   (a) If the podcast is optional: Why would they take time out of their day to listen to the podcast? What about the show is different or beneficial for their careers or education?

A rule of thumb for podcast content is to cover something that interests you, something your audience needs that excites and engages them (because the content does that for you!). Whatever you decide, the recommendation is to set clear goals with your audience. Your audience should know what to expect from your show and develop a relationship with it and you. Measuring the success of your podcast will come overtime as you watch your listenership and hear feedback from you audience on how to improve your content. In addition to engagement from your target demographic, there are evidence based metrics to help you gauge how effective your podcast is for medical education.

Universal Quality Metrics

Quality metrics are measurable indicators to help evaluate how well your podcast is performing and how much your intended audience likes the show.

There are numerous quality metrics for podcasts. The most used is something called download numbers. Download numbers measure how many times an episode is downloaded from your hosting platform. These include automatic downlands, such as when someone subscribes to your show, and manual downloads. A download number doesn't mean someone listened to your podcast, it just means the file was requested.

Another number now used to try to ascertain if someone actually listened to the show is the Interactive Advertising Bureau or IAB number. The IAB number filters out things such as bot traffic, duplicate downloads from the same user or device and downloads that don't meet a minimum duration threshold. Depending on the platform you use for your podcast, you will likely have the option to see IAB compliant downloads and non-IAB compliant downloads. Again, this is going to be a better indicator as to how engaging your content is.

As we reviewed, medical education podcasting can have intended audiences of varying sizes. Before you begin you should have some idea what the total number of your audience could be. For example, if your show is intended to be for dental students in the first and second year, that number is approximately 7000 students [6]. That means if you get 3500 downloads per episode, you may have captured 50% of the US's dental students and could consider that a success (glass half full!). Whereas if your show is created for primary care physicians,

Table 4.3 Universal quality metrics for a podcast

Metric	Description
Download numbers	Counts how often an episode file is downloaded
IAB-compliant downloads	A more accurate download count which takes into consideration bot traffic, multiple downloads, and duration of podcast that was listened to
Listener retention rate	Percentage of an episode listened to; reflects engagement in content
Completion rate	How many listeners finish an episode; key for gauging pacing and value
Subscriber growth	Change in followers or subscribers over time

there are approximately 279,000 primary care physicians in the United States [7]. If you have 3500 downloads per episode, that means at best, you captured 1.2% of the total market.

Download numbers are not the only quality metric. Table 4.3 has a list of other potential quality metrics for a podcast.

Quality Metrics for a Medical Education Podcast

The quality indictors discussed above can be used for any type of podcast, not just medical education. Now we'll discuss some quality indicators specifically for a medical education podcast.

The reason for quality indicators specific to medical education podcasts is the potential for harm if incorrect medical information is spread and propagated. This has become more relevant as more training and education programs use podcasts in their curriculum, and as more podcasts are developed under the guise of being for health and wellness.

One of the first widely used quality indicators for medical education podcasts came from a modified Delphi study in 2015 and gave us 12 items with over a 90% agreement as a necessity for a serious medical podcast [8].

After this study several quality metrics were created and modified in relation to medical podcasts. METRIQ stands for the Medical Education Translational Resources: Impact and Quality team. ALIEM AIR stands for Academic Life in Emergency Medicine (ALiEM) [9, 10]. These represent the two major quality metric system in the literature. METRIQ was further evolved into METRIQ-5 and METRIQ-8 which were revisions to the original work sourced from multiple modified Delphi processes. Feedback on the METRIQ-8 from a diverse population of students, residents and attending physicians resulted in the creation of rMETRIQ which is summarized below. ALiEM AIR was created from a discussion and revision of a group of nationally recognized educators.

This rMETRIQ scoring system is organized into three domains: content, credibility and review. It's designed to be used by any listener when evaluating a medical podcast for quality. The higher the score, the more reliable and higher quality the medical information is.

As someone is considering or is planning on creating a medical education podcast, you should use these quality indicators to make sure you're meeting all the requirements to be considered a high-quality medical education podcast.

Conclusion

If you are planning on making a medical education podcast, the structure you choose is paramount to your podcasts success. Truly understanding your audience is the key to how you will format the information you present. Know your audience size, why they would be listening to your content, and what you think is important for them to learn. While considering your audience, also consider yourself and what you are passionate about. The best podcasts have a host or guests who are interested and engaged in the material they are presenting and draw the listeners in with them. Lastly, make sure you are focused on the quality of the content you present to ensure you are always presenting evidenced based information that will further learning and enhance patient care.

References

1. Hew KF, Cheung WS. Use of Web 2.0 technologies in K-12 and higher education: the search for evidence-based practice. Educ Res Rev. 2013;9:47–64. https://doi.org/10.1016/j.edurev.2012.08.001.
2. Cooper AZ, Richards JB. Lectures for adult learners: breaking old habits in graduate medical education. Am J Med. 2017;130(3):376–81. https://doi.org/10.1016/j.amjmed.2016.11.009.
3. Matava CT, Rosen D, Siu E, Bould DM. eLearning among Canadian anesthesia residents: a survey of podcast use and content needs. BMC Med Educ. 2013;13:59. https://doi.org/10.1186/1472-6920-13-59.
4. Tarchichi TR, Szymusiak J. Attending physician's attitudes toward podcasting as a source of medical education: an exploratory study. J Contin Educ Health Prof. 2020;40(2):141. https://doi.org/10.1097/CEH.0000000000000291.
5. Cho D, Cosimini M, Espinoza J. Podcasting in medical education: a review of the literature. Korean J Med Educ. 2017;29(4):229–39. https://doi.org/10.3946/kjme.2017.69.
6. New dental schools drive increasing enrollment. https://adanews.ada.org/new-dentist/2025/june/new-dental-schools-drive-increasing-enrollment/. Accessed 30 June 2025.
7. State of the Primary Care Workforce. Published online 2024.
8. Lin M, Thoma B, Trueger NS, Ankel F, Sherbino J, Chan T. Quality indicators for blogs and podcasts used in medical education: modified Delphi consensus recommendations by an international cohort of health professions educators. Postgrad Med J. 2015;91(1080):546–50. https://doi.org/10.1136/postgradmedj-2014-133230.
9. Colmers-Gray IN, Krishnan K, Chan TM, Seth Trueger N, Paddock M, Grock A, Zaver F, Thoma B. The Revised METRIQ Score: A Quality Evaluation Tool for Online Educational Resources. AEM Educ Train. 2019;3(4):387–92. https://doi.org/10.1002/aet2.10376. PMID: 31637356; PMCID: PMC6795360.
10. Chan TM, Grock A, Paddock M, Kulasegaram K, Yarris LM, Lin M. Examining Reliability and Validity of an Online Score (ALiEM AIR) for Rating Free Open Access Medical Education Resources. Ann Emerg Med. 2016;68(6):729–35. https://doi.org/10.1016/j.annemergmed.2016.02.018. Epub 2016 Mar 29. PMID: 27033141.10.

Chapter 5
Gear

Jason Woods

Introduction

Podcasting continues to emerge as a powerful educational medium, offering flexibility, accessibility, and a personal touch to medical education. Whether delivering a case-based discussion, discussing recent research, or engaging in thought-provoking interviews, your voice becomes the primary tool through which content is delivered and received. As a medical professional stepping into podcasting, understanding the technical aspects of your setup may feel outside your comfort zone—but choosing the right gear can elevate your message, build credibility, and enhance learner engagement.

This chapter provides a practical guide to the essential hardware and software involved in podcast production. From microphones to lighting, audio interfaces to editing software, we will walk you through the considerations necessary to select tools that match your goals, environment, and budget. Our goal is not to make you an audio engineer, but to help you avoid common pitfalls and make informed decisions that allow your content to shine—clearly, professionally, and with minimal distraction.

Audio/Video Equipment

Selecting the right audio and video equipment ensures clarity and professionalism in educational content. The appropriate choice depends on factors such as budget, environment, technical expertise, and intended use. A well-thought-out setup

J. Woods (✉)
Pediatrics-Emergency Medicine, University of Colorado School of Medicine, Aurora, CO, USA

J. Parga-Belinkie et al. (eds.), *Podcasting for Medical Professionals*, https://doi.org/10.1007/978-3-032-16480-3_5

minimizes distractions, ensuring that learners focus on the educational material rather than audio or video quality. Good equipment is available no matter your budget.

When choosing audio and video equipment, educators should consider the physical space where recordings will take place (we will discuss space considerations later in this chapter). Larger lecture halls may require more powerful microphones and cameras, while small, controlled environments can benefit from simpler, more affordable options. Additionally, understanding lighting needs and audio interface capabilities ensures a polished production. Testing equipment before recording is essential to troubleshoot potential issues and ensure smooth delivery.

Choosing the Right Microphone

Audio quality is one of the most critical factors in producing professional educational content. The type of microphone chosen for recording can greatly impact the clarity and effectiveness of the final product. Different types of microphones are designed to serve specific needs, and understanding the differences between them is key to selecting the right one for your purpose.

Microphone Connection

USB Microphones

USB microphones are plug-and-play devices, making them convenient for individuals who don't have and/or need a dedicated audio interface. These microphones connect directly to a computer via a USB port, are easy to set up, usually do not require specific software to use, and are quite beginner friendly. While they are often less customizable than XLR microphones (which require an audio interface), USB mics provide convenience and ease of use. They can still offer high-quality sound, especially with models designed specifically for vocal clarity.

XLR Microphones

An XLR microphone is a microphone that uses an XLR connector, a three-pin plug commonly used in the audio industry for balanced audio signals. Historically this type of microphone provided superior sound quality with less susceptibility to noise and interference compared to USB microphones, though as technology has advanced the gap continues to shrink. Notably, XLR microphones typically require an audio interface or mixer to convert the analog signal into a digital format for recording or broadcasting. XLR microphones provide additional customizability via the associated audio interface which can often best match different individual vocal range, pitch, and dynamics. For many podcasters this customizability may not be required and the additional cost of both the microphone and the audio interface may make XLR a less desirable choice. For others the improved quality and historic reliability may be important.

Microphone Types

Condenser Microphones

Condenser microphones are highly sensitive and responsive, making them ideal for controlled recording environments such as studios or quiet rooms. Condenser microphones are known for their wide frequency response and high sensitivity. This makes them perfect for capturing the full depth of sound, including subtle tones in the human voice. However, this sensitivity means they can pick up more background noise if used in a less-than-ideal environment, such as a room with a lot of echo or external sounds. Condenser microphones may also be more sensitive to factors like moisture and humidity.

Dynamic Microphones

Dynamic microphones are much less sensitive than condenser microphones, which makes them an excellent choice for live recordings or environments with more background noise. They are generally more durable and can handle high decibels, in addition to being more resistant to environmental factors like moisture and humidity. They can also be more forgiving when it comes to less-than-perfect acoustics. However, they offer a more limited frequency response compared to condensers, so they may not capture the full richness of the voice.

Lavalier Microphones (Clip-on Microphones)

Lavalier microphones, also known as lapel mics, are small clip-on microphones that are commonly used in interviews, presentations, or on-stage performances. These microphones allow the speaker to move freely without being restricted by a handheld microphone, providing a hands-free experience. Earbuds with an in-line microphone fall into this category as far as their sound quality. The primary issue with these is they will pick up background noise extensively. For most educational podcast recordings they are not ideal, though may be required if attempting to convert a live lecture into an edited audio production for later use.

Lavalier microphones are typically omnidirectional or cardioid, meaning they capture sound from all directions or from a specific front-facing area, respectively.

They are ideal for situations where the speaker needs to be mobile, such as in video lectures or virtual classroom settings. Their small form factor makes them unobtrusive, and they can be easily clipped to clothing.

Shotgun Microphones

Shotgun microphones are designed with a very narrow pickup pattern, meaning they capture sound from a specific direction while minimizing side and rear noise. They are highly directional, making them perfect for capturing audio from a single subject or source in environments where background noise must be minimized. These tend to be used when a speaker needs to be at distance from the microphone, such as news broadcast interviews when recording on scene or in film production. They are rarely used in medical education podcasting.

Choosing Based on Directionality

Directionality refers to the pattern in which a microphone picks up sound. Microphones typically fall into the following categories based on their directionality:

- **Omnidirectional Microphones:** Capture sound equally from all directions. Ideal for situations where the speaker is moving or multiple speakers are involved, as they can pick up all surrounding sounds.
- **Cardioid Microphones:** Capture sound primarily from the front of the microphone, rejecting noise from the sides and rear. This is the most common pattern and is ideal for situations where the speaker is stationary and facing the microphone.
- **Supercardioid/Hypercardioid Microphones:** Offer even more directional sound capture than cardioid mics, with a narrower focus. These are suitable for capturing audio in environments with higher noise levels or for isolating specific sounds.
- **Figure-8 Microphones:** Capture sound from the front and rear, rejecting sound from the sides. These are often used for interviews or podcasts with two speakers, where both sides need to be picked up clearly.

Choosing Based on the Physical Environment

When selecting a microphone, it's also important to assess the space in which you'll be recording. If you are recording in a room with echo or significant ambient noise, a dynamic microphone might be more appropriate due to their noise rejection capabilities. In quieter, more controlled spaces, a condenser microphone might be the best choice for its detailed, clear sound capture. Many educational podcasters will by necessity record from their home or work offices, which have variable levels of control over echo or ambient noise, and these factors may force a decision in one direction or another. Some podcasters can alter their physical environments, installing items such as sound panels on the walls to reduce echo. For those that cannot, temporary items such as foldable sound panels or even moving pads are often adequate for podcasting needs.

One important consideration is that many consumers of spoken audio are used to listening to radio broadcasts or phone calls, where the quality of the sound and level of background noise are highly variable. As compared to sound studio recordings of music where ambient noise may be immediately noticeable and bothersome to the listener, for podcasting minor background noise or lesser vocal quality is often expected. Medical education podcasters may find that their average listener does not notice these differences, and this makes more affordable equipment or noisier environments acceptable (Fig. 5.1).

Choosing an Audio Interface or Production Console

An audio interface is a crucial component in professional audio recording setups, which typically only process sound in analog rather than digital format. Its primary function is to convert the analog signal from the microphone into a digital format that can be processed by your computer or recording software. In addition to signal conversion, audio interfaces often provide additional features such as preamps, headphone outputs, and signal routing, all of which enhance the quality and flexibility of your recordings.

When choosing an audio interface, it's important to consider the number of inputs and outputs you require. For a solo podcaster or educator, a two-input interface may be sufficient, but for more complex setups—such as recording interviews or multiple speakers simultaneously—a larger interface with more inputs and outputs will be necessary. It's also essential to evaluate the interface's compatibility

- Do you need something plug-and-play with minimal setup?
  - Yes → USB Microphone
  - No → Next question
- Are you recording more than one speaker at a time or seeking pro-level audio customization?
  - Yes → XLR Microphone with Audio Interface
  - No → USB or Lavalier Mic
- Is your environment quiet and controlled (no echo, no ambient noise)?
  - Yes → Condenser Microphone
  - No → Dynamic Microphone
- Will the speaker be moving around or standing far from the mic?
  - Yes → Lavalier or Shotgun Microphone
  - No → Stick with USB/XLR Condenser/Dynamic

Fig. 5.1 Microphone selection flowchart (beginner-friendly)

with your recording software, as well as its performance in terms of low latency and high-quality preamps.

Key Considerations in Choosing an Audio Interface

1. **Input/Output Channels:** The number of input channels determines how many microphones, instruments, or audio sources you can record simultaneously. If you plan to record multiple people at once or include instruments in your recordings, you'll need an interface with multiple inputs.
2. **Preamps:** A microphone preamp amplifies the signal from your microphone to line-level. High-quality preamps ensure clean, clear audio without distortion. Some interfaces offer built-in preamps with adjustable gain, while others may require an external preamp. The importance of the preamp may be underrated by those just entering this field, but is one of the more crucial factors in the quality of your sound recording. If the audio is not elevated to the correct gain or is not clean, all further manipulation of that audio (for instance in editing software or just turning the volume up when listening) will be affected.
3. **Sample Rate and Bit Depth:** The sample rate determines the number of samples per second your audio is captured at, while the bit depth controls the audio's dynamic range. A higher sample rate (such as 48 or 96 kHz) and bit depth (24-bit) result in clearer, more detailed audio.
4. **Latency:** Latency refers to the delay between when sound enters the microphone and when it is heard through your speakers or headphones. Low-latency interfaces are important for real-time audio monitoring (so that you are hearing exactly what the microphones are picking up at the same time they are picking it up), especially in live broadcasts or recording sessions. Many modern interfaces feature direct monitoring options, allowing you to hear the input signal without delay.
5. **Connectivity:** Many audio interfaces connect to a computer via USB, Thunderbolt, or even Wi-Fi in some cases. USB interfaces are the most common, offering wide compatibility with both Windows and macOS devices. Thunderbolt interfaces offer faster data transfer speeds, which is useful for high-track count recordings or large projects.

Types of Audio Interfaces

1. **Basic Interfaces:** These are ideal for solo recordings, podcasting, or content creation where only one or two microphones are needed. They provide the essential features for high-quality recordings, typically with minimal inputs and outputs.
2. **Advanced Interfaces:** For users who require more features or plan on recording multiple sources simultaneously, advanced interfaces offer additional channels,

premium preamps, and greater connectivity options. These interfaces are often used in professional recording studios or for live sound reinforcement.

3. **Production Consoles:** If you are looking for full control over audio production in a live or multi-source recording environment, production consoles offer extensive mixing capabilities. These consoles are typically used by larger studios or for broadcasting purposes. They allow for live sound adjustments and greater control over each audio channel.

Additional Considerations

- **Software Compatibility:** Ensure the interface you choose is compatible with your preferred recording and editing software. Most interfaces support major digital audio workstations (DAWs) like Adobe Audition, Audacity, Logic Pro, etc.
- **Portability:** If you need to record while traveling or on location, consider an interface that's compact and lightweight.
- **Monitoring Features:** Many interfaces provide headphone outputs with volume control for real-time monitoring. Some interfaces even offer zero-latency direct monitoring, which is essential for live recording.

Creating an Affordable Recording Space

While expensive studios and professional soundproofing can yield pristine audio, medical educators can achieve excellent results in makeshift or home environments with a few strategic choices. The key to recording clean, clear audio isn't always about the most expensive gear—it's often about the *space* you record in. With minimal investment, you can dramatically improve sound quality by optimizing your environment.

Room Selection

Start by choosing the quietest space available. Look for a room that:

- Has minimal outside noise (away from traffic, elevators, HVAC systems).
- Is smaller in size, with less echo or reverb.
- Has items which create less echo (soft surfaces) such as carpeted floors, curtain, bookshelves with books, pillows, and upholstered furniture.

Avoid recording in rooms with bare walls, high ceilings, or tile floors, which reflect sound and introduce unwanted echo. If you are forced to record in areas which create significant echo, sound treatment can help.

DIY Sound Treatment

You don't need professional acoustic panels to dampen sound. Many common household items work well. You may not have the option to permanently alter the space where you are recording, but many of the following can be deployed temporarily just during your recording.

- **Thick blankets or moving pads**: Hang on walls, doors, or over windows to reduce echo.
- **Closets full of clothes**: Surprisingly effective for recording—many podcasters record inside closets for their sound-dampening benefits.
- **Foldable foam or cardboard dividers**: Line them with fabric or foam and place around your mic to create a mini vocal booth.

Mic Positioning and Surfaces

- Keep your microphone off reflective or vibratory surfaces. If you can purchase a desktop arm or stand to hold your microphone, many of have vibration reducing features. If these mounts are not available, you can place a towel or small foam pad under the mic to absorb vibrations.
- Speak at a consistent distance (4–6 inches) from the mic, slightly off-axis to reduce plosives (harsh "p" and "b" sounds).
- Use a pop filter or foam windscreen, both inexpensive solutions to improve vocal clarity.

Noise Control

Turn off fans, computers, or other noisy electronics during recording. If able, do not let the HVAC system run while recording, as both the sound of the fan as well as starts/stops of the system can be highly noticeable on recording. Laptops or desktops should be positioned as far away from the mic as possible, so the sound of their fans is not picked up. Record at times when ambient noise is the lowest (traffic, coworkers, family members).

If that's not possible:

- Place laptops or desktops on foam pads or in another room and connect via a longer USB or audio cable.
- Record at times when ambient noise is lowest

Visual Considerations

Over the years many podcasters have included video content in addition to audio materials. The breadth of choices in camera features, cost, type, and quality may be even larger than for microphones. The breakdown of this extensive information is outside of the scope of this textbook. For most educators presenting primarily via podcast or as part of remote educational delivery, a standard webcam will be sufficient. For these purposes many learners are accepting of lower quality video and are used to variable quality as part of social media consumption.

Choosing a Background

When incorporating video into educational content, the background plays a crucial role in maintaining a professional and distraction-free presentation. A cluttered or chaotic backdrop can divert attention from the content, while a well-considered background enhances the viewer's focus on the speaker. Opt for backgrounds that don't overpower the speaker. A solid color wall, a tidy bookshelf, or a plant can create a clean, professional look. Avoid busy patterns or bright colors that may compete with the speaker's attire or facial features. Patterns and bright colors in the background can also sometimes cause issues when using a video conferencing platform, as the software can get confused about what is in the background versus the speaker.

If your podcast or educational content has a brand, try incorporating elements of this into the background. This could be a branded logo on the wall, consistent color schemes, or educational materials relevant to your content.

Virtual backgrounds can be helpful if you lack an ideal physical setting. Choose subtle themed visuals or neutral tones and ensure the virtual background is high-quality to avoid distracting glitches during recording. Your clothing can affect the quality of the virtual background, as if it is patterned or too similar in color to the virtual background, you may appear to be partially invisible! Test this before using in production.

Lighting

Lighting is one of the more important aspects of video capture. It can dramatically enhance or detract from the video quality, regardless of the cost or features of the camera being used. Proper lighting not only improves visibility but also sets the tone, mood, and atmosphere for the video. In educational settings, especially for medical education, good lighting can make a subject clearer, ensuring that key visual elements are properly highlighted. For these reasons, a further description of lighting is included here given its universal importance.

One important concept to consider is the difference between key lighting and fill lighting, Key lighting is the primary light source that illuminates the subject, establishing the overall look and mood of the scene. It typically comes from one direction, creating highlights and shadows that can add depth and dimension. On the other hand, fill lighting is used to reduce the shadows created by the key light, softening the contrast and providing a more balanced appearance. Fill lights are generally positioned opposite the key light (though they can also be placed below or above the speaker) and are often softer and less intense. They help ensure that facial features and important details are visible without creating harsh shadows.

Most modern lights intended for remote presentations or home video production will have companion mobile apps which provide an array of adjustments. These options may include the color (LEDs can produce near infinite shades), brightness, and temperature. Color temperature is measured in Kelvin (K), with lower values (2700–3200 K) producing warm, yellowish tones, and higher values (5000–6500 K) producing cool, bluish tones. For most video production, particularly educational content, daylight-balanced lighting (5500–6500 K) is preferred, as it mimics natural daylight and ensures a neutral, consistent look across all light sources. You will need to adjust the lights to your individual environment.

Lighting Equipment for Video Production

Natural Light

While not technically "equipment", natural sunlight can be a powerful and free lighting tool. Many spaces where you may record a podcast will have windows, and their effect can be dramatic on video quality. The sunlight should be soft and indirect, as direct sunlight can cause overexposure, sharp contrasts, or white out a portion of your face. As with the other lighting discussed here, positioning of the window in relation to your face is key. The light should be in front or off to the side (though be careful not to overexpose only one side of your face) and never behind you. Backlighting can make you appear as a silhouette, making it difficult to see your facial expressions. Timing is also important when using natural light. Early morning or late afternoon light is often the most flattering.

Softboxes

Softboxes are commonly used lighting tools in video production. They create soft, even lighting that reduces harsh shadows and highlights on the subject. By diffusing the light, softboxes help in providing a more flattering, natural look, which is important when the subject is speaking directly to the camera or giving a presentation. The larger the softbox, the softer and more even the lighting will be. This makes softboxes particularly effective for creating a balanced, neutral look for face-to-camera recordings.

LED Panels

LED panels have become popular lighting solutions for video production due to their portability, versatility, and energy efficiency. These lights emit a broad, even light that can be adjusted in terms of brightness and color temperature. LED panels are ideal for both key lighting and fill lighting, making them a valuable addition to any production setup. Their slim profile and adjustable settings make them easy to position in tight spaces, and many models are battery-powered, adding further flexibility for mobile productions.

Ring Lights
Ring lights are a popular choice for close-up shots and face-to-camera presentations. These circular lights provide even, soft lighting around the subject's face, reducing shadows and highlighting key features. Ring lights are particularly effective for creating a flattering look and are commonly used by content creators, vloggers, and educators who need to appear on screen in a polished, well-lit manner.

Practical Lights
Practical lights are lights that are visibly part of the scene, adding atmosphere or mood to the video. These can be used to create a naturalistic look, as they mimic real-world lighting, such as desk lamps, ceiling lights, or neon signs. While not the primary source of illumination, practical lights can enhance the production's visual appeal and reinforce the intended ambiance.

- **Desk Lamps with Adjustable Arms:** These can be positioned strategically in a scene to illuminate objects, documents, or the presenter in a naturalistic manner. Adjustable desk lamps are flexible and can be placed to provide dynamic, low-level lighting.
- **LED Strip Lights:** These are often used as accent lighting, adding color or texture to the background. LED strip lights can be placed along the edges of walls, shelves, or behind the subject to create an interesting visual effect.

Software

Audio editing software plays a crucial role in producing high-quality audio for medical education content, including podcasts, lectures, and recorded lessons. The right software allows you to clean up audio, adjust sound levels, remove unwanted noise, add effects, and enhance overall sound quality. Given the variety of options available, it's important to understand the key features of audio editing software and select the one that best meets your needs, whether you are a beginner, an experienced editor, or a professional sound engineer.

Key Considerations for Choosing Audio Editing Software

When selecting audio editing software for medical education content, there are several factors to consider, including the ease of use, available features, cost, and compatibility with other tools. Medical education content often requires precise audio editing, especially for instructional podcasts and video lectures where clarity is essential for learner understanding.

1. **Ease of Use and Learning Curve**

   Some audio editing programs, such as Audacity and GarageBand, are user-friendly and suitable for beginners or educators who don't have extensive experience with audio editing. These tools offer basic editing features which a user is likely already familiar with from text editing programs like cutting, trimming, and adding effects with intuitive interfaces, making them ideal for simple, fast editing tasks.

   However, more advanced software such as Adobe Audition or Hindenburg Journalist Pro offer a wider range of professional-grade features that provide more control over the sound and quality of the recording. While these tools are more powerful, they can have a steeper learning curve. If you're new to audio editing, starting with simpler software may be beneficial until you're ready to explore more complex options.
2. **Features and Tools**

   The functionality of the audio editing software is crucial, particularly for medical education. Different programs offer a variety of features depending on your editing needs. Here are some important tools and features to look for:

   - **Multi-Track Editing:** This is essential for creating any content involving more than one audio source. Multi-track editing allows you to layer different audio files, enabling you to synchronize dialogue, sound effects, and background music effectively. It also allows you to edit out mistakes in one track without affecting the others.
   - **Noise Reduction and Audio Restoration:** For medical educators, background noise can be distracting and detract from the clarity of the content. Features like noise reduction, de-essing (reduction of the prominence of sibilant consonants like s, z, ch, sh) and audio restoration can help eliminate hum, hiss, or room noise, ensuring a clean, professional sound.
   - **Equalization and Compression:** Equalization (EQ) allows you to adjust the balance of frequencies in your audio to make speech sound more natural and clearer. Compression ensures that the audio levels are consistent, preventing large volume fluctuations.
   - **Automatic Level Adjustment:** Programs like Hindenburg offer automatic level adjustment, which can be especially helpful when recording multiple speakers in varying audio conditions, ensuring consistent audio levels across tracks.
   - **Export Options:** Make sure the software supports exporting audio in various formats such as MP3, WAV, or FLAC. Having multiple export options gives you flexibility in how you distribute your content across platforms.

3. **Compatibility with Other Software**

   In a modern production environment, audio editing software is often just one part of the workflow. It's essential to choose software that integrates well with other tools you may be using, such as video editing software, podcast hosting platforms, or virtual studios. For instance, if you plan to create video content alongside your audio, ensure that your audio editing software can export in a format that works seamlessly with your video editing programs prior to making any purchases. Additionally, many audio editing programs offer support for various plugins and third-party tools. For example, Audacity supports VST plugins, allowing you to expand its functionality with additional effects, EQs, and compression tools.

4. **Budget**

   Budget is another important consideration when choosing audio editing software. Many high-quality programs, like Audacity, are free, making them ideal for individuals or institutions with limited funds. However, free software may lack some of the more advanced features available in paid programs. When evaluating software, consider whether the extra features are worth the additional cost. Many paid programs offer an extensive library of effects and premium features which are often not needed in podcast production,

5. **Support and Community**

   As with any software, support and community resources can greatly affect your user experience. A well-established community can provide valuable resources, including tutorials, troubleshooting tips, and user forums, which can help you resolve issues quickly and efficiently. Most software will have many users who have posted instructional videos on different aspects of the software.

Popular Audio Editing Software Options

Here's an overview of some of the most popular audio editing software options for medical education content creators:

1. **Audacity**

   Description: Audacity is a free, open-source audio editing software that is widely used by educators, podcasters, and musicians. It provides basic editing tools like cutting, trimming, and exporting audio in multiple formats. It's easy-to-learn interface and extensive support for plugins make it a great choice for beginners or those with minimal audio editing experience.

   Pros: Free, open-source, widely supported.

   Cons: Lacks some advanced features found in premium programs.

2. **Adobe Audition**

   Description: Adobe Audition is a professional audio editing program that offers a complete suite of features for recording, editing, and mastering audio. It is well-suited for advanced users who need powerful tools for noise reduction, sound restoration, and multi-track editing. It integrates seamlessly with other Adobe Creative Cloud tools.

Pros: Advanced features, excellent noise reduction tools, seamless integration with other Adobe products.

Cons: Subscription-based, expensive.

3. **Final Cut Pro**

   Description: Final Cut Pro is a powerful, professional video editing software designed for Mac users. It offers a comprehensive suite of tools for video editing, color grading, audio mixing, and effects, making it ideal for content creators who require precision and versatility. Final Cut Pro stands out for its magnetic timeline, efficient workflows, and seamless integration with other Apple applications.

   Pros: Powerful editing tools, intuitive interface, seamless integration with macOS, and optimized for Apple hardware.

   Cons: Only available for macOS, relatively high cost.

4. **Hindenburg Journalist Pro**

   Description: Hindenburg Journalist Pro is designed specifically for content creators who need to produce high-quality audio quickly and efficiently. It offers features like automatic leveling, noise reduction, and an intuitive interface. Its focus on storytelling and ease of use makes it an excellent choice for educators creating podcasts, interviews, or educational recordings.

   Pros: Easy-to-use interface, automatic leveling, great for podcasting.

   Cons: More limited in features compared to Adobe Audition.

5. **Reaper**

   Description: Reaper is an affordable audio editing software that offers professional features such as multi-track recording, sound restoration, and MIDI support. It has a flexible pricing model that makes it suitable for educators and content creators who need powerful tools without breaking the bank.

   Pros: Affordable, highly customizable, extensive feature set.

   Cons: Can have a steep learning curve.

6. **GarageBand**

   Description: GarageBand is a free audio editing software for Mac users. It offers a range of features suitable for beginners, including basic editing tools, multi-track recording, and a library of sound effects. While it doesn't have the advanced capabilities of software, it's a great starting point for those new to audio editing.

   Pros: Free, user-friendly, excellent for basic editing.

   Cons: Lacks some advanced features, only available for Mac users.

Hosting Platforms

Selecting the right podcast hosting platform is crucial for ensuring your medical education podcast reaches its intended audience efficiently. A podcast hosting platform stores and distributes your audio files to various podcast directories, such as Apple Podcasts, Spotify, and Google Podcasts. The hosting platform also provides essential tools for managing your content, including analytics to track your audience's engagement and automated publishing features for consistent content delivery.

Key Considerations for Choosing a Podcast Hosting Platform

When selecting a podcast hosting platform for medical education content, there are several factors to consider, including cost, ease of use, storage capabilities, analytics, and additional features that will enhance your workflow. Key elements to evaluate include:

1. **Storage and Bandwidth**
   The amount of storage and bandwidth provided by the hosting platform is essential for ensuring that your podcast runs smoothly without interruptions or limitations. Storage is important for keeping all your episodes without having to delete older content, while bandwidth ensures that your episodes can be downloaded or streamed by many listeners without crashing or causing delays. Many platforms offer unlimited bandwidth, but it's essential to verify this and choose a provider that can scale with your podcast's growth.
2. **Ease of Use and User Interface**
   The user interface of the podcast hosting platform plays a significant role in your workflow. A platform with an intuitive design makes it easier to upload, edit, and publish episodes quickly, freeing up more time for content creation and promotion. Platforms that offer drag-and-drop upload features, customizable podcast pages, and automated scheduling options can streamline the process of managing your podcast and help you maintain a consistent publishing schedule.
3. **Podcast Directories and Distribution**
   One of the primary functions of a podcast hosting platform is to distribute your content to podcast directories, including Apple Podcasts, Spotify, and Google Podcasts. When choosing a podcast hosting platform, ensure that it integrates easily with the most popular podcast directories. A good hosting platform will generate a feed for you, which is automatically updated with new episodes and sent to these directories.
4. **Analytics and Reporting**
   Analytics are essential for understanding your audience and improving the content you produce. A good podcast hosting platform should offer detailed metrics, including the number of downloads, listener demographics, listener retention rates, and geographical locations of listeners. These insights allow you to make data-driven decisions to improve your podcast, such as tailoring content to specific demographics or adjusting publishing strategies based on listener engagement.

- **Listener Metrics:** Look for a platform that provides in-depth listener metrics, such as download trends, listener demographics, episode performance, and engagement rates.
- **Retention Data:** Understanding how long listeners stay engaged with each episode is important for identifying which topics resonate the most and where listeners might lose interest. This data helps you refine your content and improve future episodes.

5. **Monetization and Sponsorship Opportunities**

   While medical education podcasts may primarily aim to inform and educate, some educators may also want to explore monetization options. Many podcast hosting platforms provide tools for monetization, such as integrating ads, offering premium subscriptions, or providing donation links. If you plan to monetize your podcast, consider choosing a platform that offers built-in monetization tools or allows you to integrate third-party tools, such as Patreon or ad networks, into your podcast.

   - **Ad Insertion:** Some platforms offer dynamic ad insertion, which automatically places ads into your podcast during editing or distribution. If monetization is important, look for platforms with this feature.
   - **Premium Subscriptions and Donations:** If you plan to offer exclusive content for paying listeners, ensure that your hosting platform supports premium subscription models or integrates with platforms like Patreon to allow listener donations.

6. **Technical Support and Customer Service**

   Having reliable technical support is essential, particularly when issues arise with hosting or distribution. Choose a platform that offers responsive customer support via email, live chat, or phone. Platforms with robust customer support can help troubleshoot issues quickly, ensuring your podcast continues to run smoothly without disruptions.

   - **24/7 Support:** Look for platforms that offer around-the-clock support in case you encounter issues with your hosting, distribution, or analytics.
   - **Community and Tutorials:** Platforms with active communities and detailed tutorials can also be helpful resources for troubleshooting and improving your podcasting process.

7. **Pricing**

   Podcast hosting platforms often offer different pricing tiers based on storage and bandwidth usage. Some platforms offer free basic plans, while others have monthly or yearly subscriptions based on the features provided. Consider the size of your podcast, how often you release episodes, and your expected audience size when selecting a pricing plan. Free plans are often limited in storage or features, while premium plans offer more extensive capabilities, such as unlimited storage, advanced analytics, and increased distribution options.

- **Free vs Paid:** While free hosting services may work for smaller podcasts, they typically have limitations such as restricted storage or ads inserted into your episodes. Paid services offer more control over your content and more features.
- **Custom Pricing Plans:** Some platforms offer custom pricing plans, depending on your specific needs, such as high-volume podcasts or specialized features. Some may even offer discounts to university faculty or educators.

Popular Podcast Hosting Platforms

1. **Libsyn (Liberated Syndication)**

   Best for: Experienced podcasters and large medical education podcasts.

   Description: Libsyn is one of the oldest and most established podcast hosting platforms, known for its reliability and advanced features. It offers a range of storage options, detailed analytics, monetization opportunities, and automatic distribution to major podcast directories.

   Pros: Unlimited bandwidth, extensive analytics, customizable podcast player, monetization tools.

   Cons: Pricing can be higher compared to other platforms, especially for higher storage plans.
2. **Buzzsprout**

   Best for: Beginners and small to medium-sized podcasts.

   Description: Buzzsprout is an easy-to-use platform with an intuitive interface, making it perfect for podcasters new to the medium. It provides simple hosting, distribution to major podcast directories, and helpful analytics. Buzzsprout also offers podcast transcription services and basic monetization options.

   Pros: Easy to use, free plan available, automatic episode distribution, high-quality analytics.

   Cons: Free plan has limitations on storage, fewer advanced features compared to some premium platforms.
3. **Podbean**

   Best for: Podcasters seeking both hosting and monetization options.

   Description: Podbean offers reliable hosting with features that support monetization, such as dynamic ad insertion and paid subscriptions. It's a great option for educators who may wish to monetize their podcasts while also having access to detailed analytics and an easy-to-navigate platform.

   Pros: Offers monetization features like ads and subscriptions, unlimited bandwidth, mobile app for managing content.

   Cons: The premium plans can be expensive, and the free plan has some storage and feature limitations.

4. **Blubrry**

   Best for: Medical education podcasters seeking detailed analytics and easy integration with WordPress.

   Description: Blueberry's podcast hosting service provides great flexibility, including powerful analytics and integration with WordPress websites. It also offers dynamic ad insertion, episode scheduling, and unlimited bandwidth, which makes it a popular choice for those with high-volume or educational podcasts.

   Pros: Excellent analytics, WordPress integration, monetization tools, no bandwidth restrictions.

   Cons: Can be difficult for beginners due to its more complex setup.

5. **Transistor**

   Best for: Professional podcasters and those needing advanced features.

   Description: Transistor is a powerful podcast hosting platform that provides unlimited storage, detailed analytics, and the ability to manage multiple podcasts from a single account. It also offers private podcast feeds for exclusive content.

   Pros: Unlimited storage, easy-to-use interface, detailed analytics, private podcast option.

   Cons: Higher cost compared to some competitors.

Websites/Feeds/Show Notes

Websites, feeds, and show notes are essential components of a robust digital content ecosystem. These elements help to structure and promote your content, making it easily accessible and providing additional value for your listeners and viewers. Websites serve as a central hub for your content, while show notes and feeds can enhance discoverability, engagement, and audience retention (Table 5.1).

Table 5.1 Podcast setup matrix

Podcast type	# of people	portability	Ideal mic setup	Other essentials
Solo, beginner	1	High	USB dynamic mic	Headphones, laptop
Interview (remote)	2+	Medium	USB mics + virtual studio	Squadcast/Zencastr, headphones
Interview (in person)	2+	Low	XLR mics + audio Interface	Headphones, foam panels, mic stands
Lecture conversion	1	High	Lavalier mic or shotgun	Audio editor for cleanup
Professional studio feel	1–4	Low	XLR mics + Interface + mixer	Pop filters, sound panels, LED lights

Websites

For medical educators producing podcasts, video lectures, or other multimedia materials, a website can be invaluable for branding, content distribution, and audience engagement. A well-designed website serves as the digital front door to your educational resources and provides a platform for potential students or learners to explore and access your materials. Wordpress and Squarespace are two commonly used website platforms, though many others exist.

When creating a website for your content, consider the following features:

- **Content Organization**: An effective website structure helps your audience navigate your content easily. Organize your materials into categories or series, whether by topic, course, or format. This structure makes it easier for learners to find specific content and follow along with your curriculum.
- **Search and Filter Functionality**: Ensure that your website includes a search function to help visitors find specific episodes, articles, or resources. Filtering options based on keywords, topics, or release dates can further enhance the user experience.
- **Mobile Optimization**: Many users access educational content through mobile devices, so your website should be responsive and mobile-friendly. This is typically a basic function of any website builder but it is worth ensuring your website looks appropriate on both desktop and mobile devices.
- **Blog Integration**: Blogging can be an excellent way to provide additional context and expand on topics discussed in your podcasts or videos. Associated show notes are often posted as a blog, while you may choose to publish additional text only blog posts depending on the extent of your educational content. Frequent posts also with SEO (search engine optimization).

Feeds

A feed is a method for syndicating your audio or video content across the web, allowing subscribers to automatically receive new content as soon as it is released. Feeds are commonly used for podcast distribution, enabling listeners to subscribe and download new episodes without having to visit a website. The feed link can be used to subscribe to your content via any podcast listening app and is required for listing your content on major platforms like Apple Podcasts or Spotify. Most podcast hosting platforms automatically generate a feed link for your content once your podcast is uploaded. You can customize the feed to include metadata like episode titles, descriptions, release dates, and cover art. The most common types of feeds for audio is RSS (Really Simple Syndication) though others exist.

Show Notes

Show notes are a vital part of your content strategy, particularly for podcasting and video content. These detailed descriptions or summaries of each episode provide listeners or viewers with essential context, making the content more accessible, searchable, and user-friendly. Well-written show notes also help to increase SEO (search engine optimization) for your content, ensuring that your podcast or video appears in relevant searches.

When writing show notes, consider including the following elements:

- **Episode Summary**: Provide a concise overview of the main points or topics discussed in the episode. This allows potential listeners or viewers to quickly assess whether the content is relevant to their needs.
- **Timestamps**: Include timestamps for key moments in the episode to help listeners or viewers jump directly to relevant sections.
- **Guest Information**: If you have a guest or collaborator on your podcast or video, include a short bio or background information. This helps build credibility and gives your audience context about the expertise of your guests.
- **Links to Resources**: Include links to any resources or studies mentioned during the episode, such as medical journals, articles, or textbooks. This is especially important in educational content, where referencing academic resources can further enhance the value of your material.

Best Practices for Websites, Feeds, and Show Notes

1. **Search Engine Optimization**: Optimizing your website, feeds, and show notes for search engines is crucial for discoverability. Use relevant keywords, provide detailed episode summaries, and include internal and external links to increase the chances of appearing in search engine results. SEO optimization will also help learners find your content more easily. Most website builders will have SEO features to assist with this.
2. **Consistency**: Consistency in your website design, content structure, and show note format ensures a professional and cohesive experience for your audience. Consistent branding across your website and episodes helps reinforce your educational message and identity. While branding is not a focus of this chapter, it is often important for individuals or groups to show their content is coming from a consistent source with reliable quality.
3. **Engagement**: Encourage audience interaction by allowing for comments, reviews, or questions related to each episode. Engaging with your audience in this way creates a sense of community and encourages repeat visits or listens. Similar engagement can happen using a variety of social media platforms. Most websites allow for comment review to avoid spam or unprofessional comments on your episodes.

4. **Analytics**: Use analytics tools like Google Analytics, FeedBurner, or podcast-specific platforms to track your audience's engagement and behavior. Understanding which episodes or topics are most popular can help inform future content creation and distribution strategies. These data may also be useful for university faculty promotion.

Use of Podcast Hosting Platform Instead of a Website

Podcast hosting platforms offer tools specifically designed to help podcasters manage, organize, and distribute their show notes effectively. These platforms serve as centralized locations for managing episodes and the associated content, including show notes. For medical educators looking to streamline the process of delivering accessible, professional show notes, using the features provided by these podcast hosts can significantly reduce the technology barriers to to publication which are associated with a website.

Key Features of Podcast Hosting Platforms for Show Notes

1. **Episode-Level Show Notes**
   Many podcast hosting platforms allow users to add detailed show notes directly at the episode level. This ensures that every episode has all relevant information in one place, similar to show notes published as a blog post using a website.
2. **Customizable Show Notes Templates**
   Many of these platforms allow users to create customizable templates for their show notes. This is particularly useful for content creators who publish multiple episodes and want to maintain consistency across their show notes.
3. **SEO-Friendly Features**
   Although podcast hosting platforms are not full-fledged website builders, many of them provide SEO-friendly options to increase discoverability. Show notes are often indexed by search engines, meaning the detailed descriptions and keywords included in your episodes can help attract more listeners through organic search. Using relevant keywords and detailed descriptions can help your podcast appear in search results for users searching for specific medical topics or episodes.
4. **Podcast Aggregator Integration**
   Podcast hosting platforms generally integrate seamlessly with popular podcast directories, such as Apple Podcasts, Spotify, Google Podcasts, and more. This means that the show notes you create on your hosting platform will automatically be included in the episode description across these platforms, ensuring your content is easily accessible to a wider audience.

5. **Automatic Episode Updates**

   Many podcast hosting platforms allow for automatic updates to show notes. This is helpful when new information becomes available or corrections need to be made. Medical educators can easily update their show notes to reflect new guidelines, research, or follow-up discussions without the need to revise multiple pages or platforms manually.

Virtual Studios

Virtual studios are an increasingly popular tool for creating professional-quality video content without the need for a traditional, physical studio space. In the realm of audio-focused virtual studios, the emphasis is on creating high-quality, clear audio for remote recordings, podcasts, and virtual interviews, without the need for a traditional studio setup. Virtual audio studios allow educators, podcasters, and content creators to produce professional-grade audio in a controlled, remote environment, using cloud-based software that mimics the features of an in-person audio recording studio. These platforms typically offer advanced audio mixing and noise reduction. More importantly, most offer multi-track recording, meaning each participant's voice is recorded separately, allowing for better post-production editing and ensuring that background noise or technical issues with one participant don't affect the entire recording. Virtual studios may also offer the ability to edit your tracks directly in their platforms instead of moving to other software. Some creators may enjoy this streamlining though many may feel the results of their editing are better in dedicated audio editing software.

Here are some popular audio-focused virtual studio platforms:

- **Squadcast**: Squadcast is an excellent tool for remote podcast recording and creating high quality audio. It provides automatic backup recording in case of connectivity issues and offers high-fidelity lossless audio recordings.
- **Zencaster**: Zencaster is another web-based platform very similar to Squadcast with equivalent features. These two platforms vary over time in pricing and often the choice between one or the other depends on cost.
- **Riverside**: Riverside is a cloud-based recording platform tailored for both audio and video production. It is particularly useful when you want to create a video companion to your podcast. Anywhere, and each track is recorded locally to ensure the highest possible audio quality.
- **Streamyard**: Although Streamyard is typically associated with live video streaming, it also offers excellent audio-focused features for podcasting and features similar to Riverside.

Key Features to Look for in Audio-Focused Virtual Studios

1. **Multi-Track Recording**: Look for virtual studio platforms that offer separate tracks for each participant. This allows for precise control during editing, including adjusting the gain for each track individually and editing out mistakes from one track without affecting the entire recording.
2. **High-Quality Audio**: Ensure the platform supports high-definition, lossless audio recording. Some of the higher-level platforms even offer 48 or 96 kHz recording capabilities, which are ideal for professional audio production.
3. **Noise Reduction and Audio Enhancements**: Many virtual studio platforms offer tools for real-time noise reduction, sound enhancement, and automatic audio correction. These features help to eliminate unwanted background noise, hum, or echoes, ensuring a clean, professional sound. You may decide you do not want the virtual studio platform to do this processing and you would rather do this in your audio editing software, but it's nice to have the option.
4. **Cloud-Based Storage**: Cloud-based storage is crucial for easy collaboration and access to recordings from multiple locations. Importantly, storing the recordings in the cloud *as they are created* rather than on each participants local computers reduces the possibility a tech failure on one participants computer renders the entire recording defective.
5. **Integration with Other Software**: This should be available on any widely used virtual studio, but ensure the platform will export your files into a format usable by your editing software.

Conclusion

High-quality content begins with clear, consistent audio. As medical educators, your expertise is invaluable—but without the setup, your message may lose impact or be undermined by avoidable distractions. Fortunately, the podcasting landscape now offers a range of equipment and tools to fit nearly every need and budget, from simple USB microphones for solo recordings to more advanced setups for multi-speaker interviews and video integration.

While the gear may seem secondary to your content, it plays a critical role in how that content is received. Take the time to test, iterate, and adapt based on your environment and your audience. With thoughtful investment—of time, not just money—you can build a setup that supports your teaching and reflects the professionalism your learners expect.

Bibliography

1. Brown A, Green T. The essentials of instructional design: connecting fundamental principles with process and practice. Routledge; 2020.
2. Katz B. Mastering audio: the art and the science. 3rd ed. Focal Press; 2015.
3. Koumi J. Designing video and multimedia for open and flexible learning. Routledge; 2006.
4. Mayer RE. Multimedia learning. Cambridge University Press; 2021.
5. McElroy J, McElroy T. Everybody has a podcast (except you): a how-to guide from the first family of podcasting. Harper Perennial; 2021.
6. Rode J. Podcasting made simple: the step-by-step guide. Simple Media; 2021.
7. Wouters P, van Oostendorp H. Instructional techniques to facilitate learning and motivation. Springer; 2017.

Chapter 6
Content Creation

Joanna Parga-Belinkie

Knowing Your Mission and Audience

When developing content for a medical podcast it is important to have a mission statement or a goal for the podcast. Most people decide to start a podcast because they see a problem in medicine. The problem could be there is no accessible information on a topic, or that there are so many medical advances in a field it's hard to keep up with them. The scope and solutions to that problem could also vary greatly. Generally there are two broad categories of podcasts: those that are patient facing, and those geared towards health care professionals. For patient facing podcasts, typically the goal is to educate families regarding preventative health measure, help them better understand diseases processes, or allow for community surrounding a more rare disease or pediatric health concern [1]. For health care professionals the reasons can be more varied but may center around educating other health care professionals, or again forming community around a pediatric health topic [2]. Whatever your motivations, podcasts with a central theme will likely be more successful as they will attract a specific audience with a vested interest in the topic.

Knowing the audience and in particular its size and demographics (i.e. age, race/ethnicity, level of education, geographic location etc.) will guide how you will speak to them when you are constructing content. Successful podcasts often have consistent hosts (more on that below) that can relate to their listeners and set the tone for the recording. Consider when you are talking to families the phrases you use and resources you offer will be different than when you are speaking to another healthcare professional. Table 6.1 summaries considerations for speaking with patients versus other health care professionals.

J. Parga-Belinkie (✉)
Department of Neonatology, Children's Hospital of Philadelphia, Philadelphia, PA, USA
e-mail: pargabelij@chop.edu

J. Parga-Belinkie et al. (eds.), *Podcasting for Medical Professionals*,
https://doi.org/10.1007/978-3-032-16480-3_6

Table 6.1 Strategies for effective communication tailored to your podcast audience

Audience	Communication strategies
Families/Patients	Avoid medical jargon Consider a sixth grade reading level for inclusivity Adopt a conversational and less of a professorial tone
Health Care Professionals	Ok to use medical terminology Can consider a higher reading level (ie college or graduate level) when scripting material May be responsive to more lecture-based content
Universal Audience Considerations	Consider translating materials into different languages based on listenership Use stories/clinical vigenettes when possible to engage the listener

Any medical professional can consider starting a podcast because the dissemination of evidence-based content in approachable formats is needed in our unregulated, information dense society [3]. Additionally there is minimal technical know-how required for podcasting and putting out audio content. That said, even when a specific need and audience are identified, it is important to know what other podcasts exist in your niche before writing or recording. Not only will this give you insights in how to differentiate your podcast, but it will also give you a list of potential collaborators for your work. The podcasting community thrives on shared visions and goals. The hope is your podcast will add something unique to the discourse around your topic, something that differentiates it from what is already heard by your audience.

Thought Exercises to Engage in Before Starting a Medical Podcast

- **What is the gap in knowledge or problem that I am trying to address?**
  - Research what other podcasts exists in your area of interest
  - Determine what your podcast adds to exisiting content
- **Who is my audience?**
  - Determine if your audience is patients or other health care professionals Tailor language and content to this audience
  - Try to envision who your dedicated listeners will be (ie. size, race/ethnicity, level of education, geographic location)
- **Who are potential collaborators for my work?**
  - When you find similar podcasts—consider how you can work together to amplify your voices and make sure your content is evidence-based and disseminated

Structuring Your Content

You have thought about what you want to say and who you want to say it to. You've researched other podcasts in your area of interest and identified how yours will be different. It's time to start thinking about the structure of your podcast (see Chap. 4 for more details). As you imagine the structure, pieces of it that will influence your content creation include identifying who your host will be, preparing scripts for your episodes, and if conducting interviews, prepping guests to record with you.

Determining Your Host

The host of a podcast should be consistent to allow listeners to form a parasocial relationship with them [4]. This will increase listener engagement by making them feel connected to the host. There are no set qualifications needed to host a medical podcast, however, an enthusiasm for and understanding of the topic facilitates discussion and engagement. The host will be the voice of your podcast and will have a large role in shaping the content you release. Make sure this person is creative, adaptable, and agrees with the mission statement you have for your podcast (see Chap. 7 for more details on hosting).

Scripting Your Episodes

There are two approaches to preparing a script for your episode. One is to write out everything you are going to say in a full transcript of the podcast. The other is to script talking points of information you want to cover. There are pros and cons to each of these scripting techniques.

Many podcasts do rely on a script to introduce their podcast that gives the title, hosts name, and mission of the podcast [5]. This can be prerecorded and added to the beginning of all your podcast episodes. Some hosts also desire to script out all the episode prior to recording. This allows them to construct a narrative, determine the flow of the show, and have more control over the direction of the episode. Some may find this helps to organize their thoughts and decrease their anxiety about recording. This technique can be used for hosts who are monologuing their content. It can also help structure an interview by allowing for a thoughtout introduction and outro for the episode—and questions that guide you through the episode in a predictable fashion. The challenge with this type of scripting is that listeners may be able to hear that you are reading instead of adopting a more conversational tone with them. This may make the podcast sound more like a lecture, making it dry and less engaging. To help make the podcast sound more organic, imagine you are speaking directly to your listeners when you record. Emphasize parts of the script you feel are important, and allow yourself to get emotional about the content when it calls for a reaction.

Alternatively, when scripting talking points the goal is to remind yourself of the content you want to cover. It allows for a blueprint of ideas, and more flexibility in how you structure your overall episode. Hosts may find this allows for a more colloquial tone and style. Without a formal script there is also room for more spontaneity in delivery. An advantage to this from of scripting is it allows the host and guests to prioritize connection over perfection, and could lead to increased engagement in the content. A disadvantage is there is less control over the message, and important talking points might inadvertently be left out of the episode as discussion ensues or the host follows a different train of thought then they intended (Table 6.2).

When creating content—consider a spreadsheet that includes: anticipated recording topic ideas, and tentative podcast launch dates. Keep this as a living document allows you to catalogue what content you have already covered, and think of what scripting will need to be done.

Preparing Guests to Come on Your Podcast

Interview-based episodes are always a fun endeavor. It could also be what you decide is best for all your episodes depending on your mission and intended reach. Part of the joy of interviews is the ability to connect with others on a topic you care about, and extending your listenership by drawing an audience interested in what your invited guest has to say. Or just people who want to hear that guest speak.

For interviews, you want to approach the person you would like to have on your podcast with what your podcast structure is, and with a specific ask for them to speak about. Consider creating a form email that introduces you, your podcast, and then create a personalized invitation for the guest. Tell them why you thought of them for a particular topic, who your audience is, and what impact their voice would have for your listeners.

Table 6.2 Pros and cons to different scripting approaches

Scripting approach	Advantages	Disadvantages
Write out everything you want to say	More control over the message Can help decrease anxiety of what to say Will not forget important pearls or messages you want to deliver to your audience	May sound like you are reading Can come off to the listener as more of a lecture than a podcast Doesn't allow for spontaneity
Rely on talking/bullet points	Flexibility in what you cover Less prep time Facilitates conversation	Less structure Might leave out talking/bullet points

If your guests accepts an invitation to your podcast be prepared to give them two things: technical instructions on how to set up their audio recording, and tips on how to prepare the content they will discuss on the episode.

Guest Technical Instructions

Your invited guests do not need professional podcast setups to give you good audio. Headphones are an essential tool for recording, and most guests will have either wireless or wired headphones they can attach to where they record. Most will be recording either on a desktop or laptop computer, but a smartphone also can easily be used for recordings as most recording platforms have online interfaces or apps that can be accessed. Headphones are needed because if the guest does not have a microphone and are using a computer or cell phone recorder it will ensure your voice is not on their recording. This will greatly ease your editing later on by ensuring their voice is on it's own audio tract without interference from yours. Having a microphone—and it can be one built into the headphones—is also helpful to capture pure audio and reduce outside noises. Ensure your guest has a quiet place to record, preferably one where sound waves can't bounce around. Sound waves like to reverberate off of hard surfaces like wood floors and walls. That is why recording in a bedroom with lots of pillows and carpeting, or in a closet with lots of clothes will help capture sound waves so they don't bounce off each other. So ask that your guest find a quiet cozy padded place to sit down. Many for medical recordings may be in their offices, so make sure that office is one with a closed door and is not in an open space or a cubby.

Guest instructions should be clear and concise, and when scheduling an interview account for about 15 minutes or so of time to be spent on addressing technology issues to ensure quality recordings. A sample guest instructions can be seen in Box 6.1.

Box 6.1 Sample Podcast Guest Instructions (Adapted from the American Academy of Pediatrics Podcast: Pediatrician on Call Guest Intructions)

- The three most important things for getting good sound on your side are the location you record in, using headphones and having a good mic. (Ear buds you use for your phone qualify as both headphones and a mic)
- Find a quiet room to record in. (Try to avoid an echoey room, open windows or sitting near large windows with street noise. Examples: A great location would be a carpeted room with soft surfaces—like a closet. An awful location would be a hotel lobby or room with lots of hard surfaces and or high ceilings)
- Record using a computer as able. (If you need to use a phone, download the appropriate recording app)
- As able, put your phone on airplane mode to disable interruptions from other calls or notifications.
- Turn off radios, TVs, fans. Disconnect from any VPNs.
- Don't multitask while recording. Typing and sounds from software can be picked up by a mic.
- Watch for possible noise from things like bumping the table/desk or computer, clicking a pen, or banging jewelry. (It's best to remove jewelry like a bracelet or dangling earrings.)
- Please put pets in another room.
- Close email programs or anything that can make sound.
- If you make a mistake or want to restate something, you can because it will be edited. Please pause a second if you do.
- It's a conversational tone, not NPR, so relax and enjoy the interview!:)

If you are aiming for around a 30 minute recording, likely your interview time slots should be 45 minutes to 60 minutes. This will allow for you to have around 15 minutes to troubleshoot if needed, and 30 minutes to get good quality conversation recorded. If the recording takes a shorter amount of time, no one will mind ending early. If the recording time goes over, you might lose your guest to other responsibilities or appointments. Be sure to contact guests with at least one to two weeks time to plan and schedule.

Helping Your Guest Prepare Content

After giving clear instructions on how and where to record, consider if you want to give your guests the scripted interview questions you may prepare. Many guests will be curious about how to research for the interview, and giving them questions is a way for them to formulate either their own script or talking points. The disadvantage of giving out the interview questions before the recording is that it may sound staged or like a rehearsed talk instead of a spontaneous podcast conversation. Instead of providing the questions, you can consider just coaching your guest on how to prepare. Let them know what sources or articles you thought were important about the topic and inspired you. Be specific about what you hope they will discuss based on their expertise and past experiences. Ultimately you may need to just reassure your guests that when they come on a podcast—unlike live radio—is a forgiving art. It is meant to be edited, and you can ensure that when an answer is not to their liking or doesn't convey the message they intended, you can cut that segment or rework it. Assure them that they don't want to sound too rehearsed, and that you will capture their voice and their message authentically. This will help you establish rapport and allow for your guest to be mindful and sincere in their answers to your questions.

Let This Be Your Creative Spark

Now that you have an idea of how to create content—starting doing it! It can be as simple as pulling up a word document and thinking about what in medicine makes you excited, and what audience you'd like to speak to. Start a spreadsheet of podcasts you admire, topic ideas, and guests you would love to talk to. One of the delights of podcasting is that it is accessible. Even if you can't purchase fancy equipment, or get a producer or sound designer to sign on—you can still podcast. Just having a computer or phone and headphones means you have the equipment you need. Let this chapter be the spark that ignites your creativity. Your ideas and dedication to your message are the only things you need to drive your podcast creation. If making a whole podcast is not your goal, use this chapter to pitch a podcast episode to a medical podcast doing work you enjoy. That might be enough to get you invited as a guest, and you'll already know some of the rules for best engagement when you join onto a podcast that is already recording. Your voice as a medical educator and expert is so needed, so use it.

References

1. Robins B, Delaney T, Maher C, Singh B. Podcasts as a tool for promoting health-related behaviours: a scoping review. Digit Health. 2024;10(January):20552076241288630.
2. Zhang E, Trad N, Corty R, Zohrob D, Trivedi S, Rodman A. How podcasts teach: a comprehensive analysis of the didactic methods of the top hundred medical podcasts. Med Teach. 2022;44(10):1146–50.
3. Berk J, Watto M, Williams P. Twelve tips for creating a medical education podcast. Med Teach. 2020;42(11):1221–7.
4. Horton D, Wohl RR. Mass communication and para-social interaction: observations on intimacy at a distance. Psychiatry. 1956;19(3):215–29. Retrieved from https://ia802306.us.archive.org/10/items/donald-horton-and-richard-wohl-1956/Donald%20Horton%20and%20Richard%20Wohl%201956.pdf.
5. Sotério C, Queiroz SL. Improving writing skills through scripting a science podcast for non-expert audiences. J Coll Sci Teach. 2023; https://doi.org/10.1080/0047231x.2023.12315864.

Chapter 7
Being a Host

Megan Felicity Hoang and Tony Tarchichi

Introduction

A comprehensive understanding of the role of a podcast host is essential to producing and developing evidence-based medical podcasts. The host functions as an educator, communicator, narrator, researcher, and entertainer. A key determinant of a high-quality podcast is the host's ability to navigate diverse guest perspectives by adapting to the tone and pacing of real-time conversations while sustaining audience engagement. Most importantly, hosts serve as a bridge, translating complex knowledge into accessible narratives that your audience can easily understand. This chapter provides a foundation for developing strong skills as a host and offers techniques to enhance audience engagement, establish credibility, and build a meaningful presence in a medical education podcast.

M. F. Hoang (✉)
University of Pittsburgh School of Medicine, Medical Scientist Training Program, University of Pittsburgh, Pittsburgh, PA, USA
e-mail: hoang.megan@pitt.edu

T. Tarchichi
University of Pittsburgh School of Medicine. UPMC Children's Hospital of Pittsburgh – Paul C. Gaffney Division of Pediatric Hospital Medicine, Pittsburgh, PA, USA

J. Parga-Belinkie et al. (eds.), *Podcasting for Medical Professionals*,
https://doi.org/10.1007/978-3-032-16480-3_7

Interview Skills

The Art of Storytelling

Many students and residents prefer podcasts over other learning modalities because they offer practical knowledge and real-world experience through interviews and discussions with guests in addition to factual knowledge [1–3]. Hosts play a pivotal role in shaping the success of a podcast through a narrative format of communication by setting the tone, pace, and theme, while building connections with guests. This conversational style naturally lends itself to storytelling, where a host can transform any topic, even technical and complex topics into compelling narratives that resonate with a broad audience [1]. Through this artform, the brains of speakers and listeners can synchronize in a phenomenon called *neural coupling* [4]. This mirroring allows audiences to better understand and internalize the speaker's experiences. Unlike presentations centered around facts and evidence that mainly activate language-processing centers, stories stimulate multiple areas of the brain, including those involved in emotions and sensory and motor experiences [2, 5]. This multi-sensory activation makes learning richer and more enduring. In the context of medical education, where complex and abstract concepts are common, storytelling plays a crucial role. By weaving clinical data into narratives, such as patient journeys, diagnostic challenges, or experiences, podcast hosts can bridge the gap between academic knowledge and practical understanding.

Techniques for Effective Storytelling

While the benefits of storytelling are well established, mastering storytelling requires intention, structure, and practice. When presenting data from scientific papers and experimental findings, podcast hosts should weave narrative elements into these discussions. Below are foundational techniques that podcast hosts can use to elevate the quality of their interviews and engage listeners on a deeper level.

1. *Structure Interviews as Narratives*
   By framing interviews as stories, hosts can create meaningful connections with their audience that resonate across different cultures and make listeners feel understood and inspired. Strong interviews have a clear beginning, middle, and end, woven around an overarching message. Treat each interview not as a Q&A session, but as a narrative arc with a beginning, middle, and end. Consider these questions: *What is the story I am trying to help the guest tell?* Whether it's the evolution of a scientific idea, a patient's unique case, or a mentor's professional path, framing the conversation within a narrative structure helps listeners follow along and stay emotionally engaged.

   - **Beginning**: Set the stage: Introduce the guest(s), the setting (clinic, lab, etc.), and the challenge or question at hand.

- **Middle**: Explore turning points, surprises, or conflicts that make the story dynamic.
- **End**: Summarize the main findings and reflect on lessons learned and opportunities for further exploration. Leave your audience with a takeaway or challenge, something to reflect on or act upon. This final step deepens retention while reinforcing the main message and moves your audience from passive listeners to engaged participants.

2. *Use Stories as Hooks*

Start episodes with a compelling story to immediately capture attention. A well-chosen anecdote or rhetorical questions can act as a *hook*, drawing the listener in before delving into technical content. These short stories (ideally under 2 min) should introduce a relatable moment, a tension point, or an unexpected twist.

Tip: Think about your core content first, then work backward to create or choose a story that introduces the theme. Don't force the story- let it complement the educational objective.

3. *Foster Emotional Connection*

To achieve this, hosts need to go beyond presenting facts and evidence but create emotional connections with interviewees and the public. While teaching content, ask guests about their emotions, motivations, and reflections. How did they feel when they made a difficult decision? What kept them going during setbacks? By inviting vulnerability and authenticity, hosts help listeners connect with both the content and the speaker.

4. *Show, Don't Tell*

Avoid generic descriptions. Use vivid imagery and sensory details to paint a picture. Instead of saying, *"It was a stressful night in the ICU,"* say, *"The alarms wouldn't stop, the hallway lights flickered, and I hadn't eaten in 13 hours when the fourth trauma came through the doors."* These details activate the listener's imagination and make the story unforgettable.

5. *Recap and Reflect*

After a guest shares an impactful story, take a moment to reflect or reframe it for your audience. This serves two purposes: it reinforces key points and creates a connection point between the listener and the content.

6. *Master the Sound of Storytelling*

Subtle variations in a narrator's voice, such as pitch, pace, and rhythm, can significantly influence the tone of a conversation [6]. A good storyteller knows when to smile, pause, and laugh, and when to emphasize key words or moments. Avoid being uniformly loud and instead, vary your tone to match the energy of the moment. Your vocal pacing should match the emotional rhythm of the story you or your guest are telling. Mirroring your guests' communication style through language, tone, and cadence increases trust. Through careful pacing and thoughtful questions, the audience can engage with the podcast, which can increase their memory of the podcast [7]. A captivating storyteller brings confidence and energy into people to keep the audience engaged.

Audience-Centered Communication

One of the strengths of podcasting is the ability to connect people from remote locations to build a community. When hosting a medical podcast, it can be easy to focus on delivering high-quality content and worrying about whether interviews with guests run smoothly. But even the most insightful conversations can lose their impact if the audience cannot connect with the speakers and the content. It has been reported that medical residents have perceived entertainment value and listener engagement as key drivers of sustained interest in podcasts [3]. Even when covering important topics, podcasts described as monotonous or overly scripted were more likely to be abandoned by learners. Thus, it is equally important to consider how the information is presented and be cognizant of the audience listening to the podcast. Effective podcasts are not just about the host and the speaker, but also the listeners.

In a qualitative study, medical residents preferred humor and banter exchanged between hosts and guests [3]. These informal elements foster a sense of familiarity and connectedness, making the listening experience feel more personal and less isolating. Whether you are interviewing a surgeon about trauma protocols or discussing new guidelines in autoinflammatory disease, the goal of the podcast is not simply to convey information, but to guide your audience through a meaningful conversation that is relevant, accessible, and engaging. Podcasts hosts should adopt an audience-centered mindset: asking not only "What do I want to say?" but also "What does my audience want to hear, and how do they want to hear it?" This includes incorporating humor, storytelling, and moments of reflection, which help transform passive listening into active engagement. To achieve this, ask yourself: Is your conversation centering the speaker, the content, or the audience?

Let's explore the differences—starting with the speaker-centered approach.

A **speaker-centered** presentation is a one-way communication format, where the speaker (guests or host) dominates the episode, focusing primarily on their own ideas, voice, and expertise (Table 7.1). This style lacks interaction and often overlooks the needs and perspectives of the audience. As a result, listeners may feel disconnected and eventually tune out of the presentation. For example, imagine an acclaimed cardiac surgeon specialized in valve replacements giving a talk on advanced techniques in aortic valve replacement, but presenting it as a list of procedural steps and personal preferences, without offering real-world clinical scenarios, explaining the rationale behind their approach, or incorporating stories about challenges faced in the operating room or during postoperative care. While the information may be technically accurate, the lack of relatable context or narrative structure makes it difficult for the audience to connect with or apply the material. Without attention to the learners' perspective, the presentation ultimately falls flat.

Table 7.1 Speaker-Centered vs. Audience-Centered Podcast Communication

Feature	Speaker-Centered Approach	Audience-Centered Approach
Primary Focus	Speaker's expertise and message	Audience's needs, interests, and understanding
Goal	Deliver expertise	Create a meaningful, engaging learning experience
Communication Style	One-way, lecture-like	Interactive, conversational
Tone	Formal, scripted	Relatable, conversational, involves improvisation, humor, or banter
Role Of the Host	Expert or passive moderator	Active facilitator and bridge between guest and audience
Examples	Technical monologue with step-by-step details of aortic valve replacement without clinical storytelling or engagement	Includes patient cases and walks through decision-making in aortic valve replacement with audience, inviting input and explaining rationale for each choice
Common Pitfall	Overloading content without audience context	May risk oversimplification, but maintains connection
Success Indicators	Accuracy, prestige of guest	Listener retention, feedback, emotional and cognitive engagement

In contrast, **audience-centric presentation** begins with a simple but powerful question: *"What would my audience want to know next?"* This approach involves translating complex or dense expert responses into accessible, applicable insights (Table 7.1). Rather than overwhelming the listener with information, a skilled host acts as a bridge between the expert and the audience by guiding the conversation to meet the listener's level of knowledge and curiosity.

A good host is a bridge between the expert and the listener:

- Asking clarifying questions where the listener might be too shy or too new to ask
- Shaping pacing so that the audience can follow
- Pausing to reflect, summarize, or personalize

Think of it like this: the guest provides the depth, the host provides the direction, and the audience is the purpose (Fig. 7.1).

An effective host does this by:

1. *Knowing the audience beyond demographics*

Sure, your audience may be pediatric residents, but that's just the surface. Dig deeper and understand: why is your audience listening? Understanding what your audience hopes to gain or what excites them allows you to tailor your content more effectively. Even if it's because your podcast is part of a required medical school curriculum, that insight is valuable. For example, if a medical school includes your podcast episode— "Managing Acute Chest Pain in the Emergency department"—as required listening, students are tuning in because it's on the syllabus and therefore are captive but not necessarily engaged.

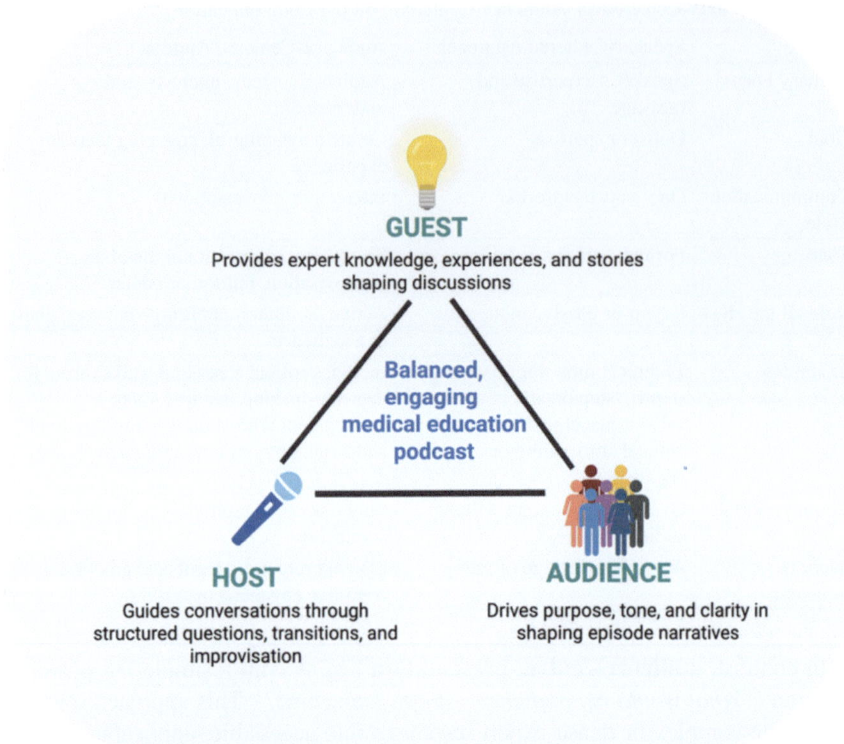
GUEST
Provides expert knowledge, experiences, and stories shaping discussions
Balanced, engaging medical education podcast
HOST
Guides conversations through structured questions, transitions, and improvisation
AUDIENCE
Drives purpose, tone, and clarity in shaping episode narratives

Fig. 7.1 The Podcast Triangle: Guest—Host—Audience. (*Created using* Biorender.com)

So what do you do?

- **Open with a hook:** Instead of diving straight into clinical jargon, begin with a gripping real case: *"A 38-year-old woman walks into the ED, clutching her chest. She's healthy. No risk factors. What do you do?"*
- **Layer in storytelling and reflection:** After explaining the management steps, bring in a cardiologist to reflect on diagnostic pitfalls or emotional moments from the cath lab. Use clear, straightforward language and avoid unnecessary complexity. Take time to explain any medical or scientific jargon or technical concepts.
- **Include pause-and-recall moments:** Every 5–7 min, insert quick recaps or questions: *"Okay, quick check—what are the three must-not-miss causes of chest pain in young adults?"*

By recognizing that your audience is there out of obligation, you can respect their time and capture their attention with engaging elements, so the information sticks with them.

2. *Understanding your audience:*

Tailor your content to the audience. For example, if there is a diverse mix of physicians and medical students, create a balance of questions that would relate to both audiences. Do your listeners want short and straight to the point episodes or narrative storytelling? Do they prefer case-based learning or reflection? Adjusting the pacing of the conversation so listeners have time to absorb and process the discussion. Effective strategies can also include verbal repetition, pause to reflect, retrieval practice, and summarize key points. Connecting the discussion to real-world practice or patient care can help solidify understanding and make your podcast more memorable and impactful.

3. *Create personal connection*

Throughout the episode, hosts should remember that they are speaking to real people rather than simply broadcasting stories and facts. Unlike live lectures, it is not possible to observe facial expressions or hear reactions from the audience. As a result, messages must be delivered with intentionality and with careful consideration of how the language and tone may be received.

Phrases such as "Some may be wondering…" or "maybe you've experienced this too" can foster a sense of personal connection, even in the absence of real-time feedback. Connect with listeners by addressing questions they might have, such as "What are common challenges or misconceptions?" or "What advice would you give to your younger self?" Referring to listener-submitted questions, previous feedback, or takeaways from earlier episodes can further cultivate a sense of inclusion and engagement. Referencing listener questions, feedback, or previous episode takeaways helps listeners feel seen and involved. Lastly, it is critical to ending the podcast with a call-to-action or tangible steps in which the audience can reflect on or apply to their persona or professional life. This allows the podcast to become more than just something they listen to—it becomes something of which they feel a part.

4. *Receive feedback*

At the end of each episode, it is important to invite listeners to share their thoughts about their listening experience. Feedback is one of the most powerful tools for growth by learning how to improve the production in future episodes and connect with your community.

Encourage your audience to respond through structured tools like polls and surveys, or through more informal channels such as episode comments and social media interactions. In surveys, consider using rating scales to assess aspects like timing, episode structure, speaker engagement, and overall clarity. Include open-ended questions in surveys, allowing listeners to elaborate on what they found most valuable, what was confusing or less engaging, and which topics or guest speakers they would like to hear in future episodes. This not only demonstrates that you value their input but also fosters a sense of community and collaboration. When receiving feedback, especially in comment sections, take the time to thank respondents, whether their input is positive or constructive. If someone offers critical feedback, respond professionally and with curiosity. However, if a comment is inappropriate or disrespectful, it's best to ignore it and focus on helpful responses.

Use the feedback you receive to identify patterns and actionable insights. Let the data inform how you shape future interviews and content structures. Do not treat feedback as a one-time occurrence but continue to integrate feedback loops throughout your podcasting process. Remind listeners at various points to share their input and act on it visibly so they feel heard. Over time, this creates a cycle of continuous improvement that both strengthens your hosting skills and ensures your podcast remains relevant, audience-centered, and impactful.

Active Listening

Podcasts in academia are built around interviews and conversations that involve active listening, which includes demonstrating non-verbal engagement with the speaker, paraphrasing to reflect the speaker's message, and probing questions to seek clarification or elaboration.

Active listening is another important technique that allows for rich and authentic discussions when speaking to guests . Beyond nodding and responding to guests' stories, hosts must be fully present during the interview to focus on what the guest is saying rather than preparing next questions. Active listening creates an environment of trust with the audience that can with nuggets and clinical pearls. Below are tips to engage in active listening throughout the episode.

1. *Pay attention and show that you are listening*
   In audio-only formats, non-verbal cues like nodding or eye contact are lost within the audience. However, engagement can still be conveyed through vocal cues—pauses, affirmations ("I see," "That's interesting"), and tone. Stay mentally present. Listen attentively without immediate judgment or interruption. This creates an atmosphere based on trust, making guests feel more comfortable sharing nuanced information, clinical pearls, and even professional vulnerabilities. Avoid thinking ahead to your next question while the guest is speaking. Instead, fully absorb their message to uncover the real substance of their story.

   - **Tip:** Listen as if watching a video. Imagine every word as a visual story unfolding to help maintain a sense of presence and immersion.

2. *Summarize and build*

Active listening involves understanding what the speaker said by summarizing and paraphrasing what was said to validate the speaker's perspective. When the guest is finished speaking, paraphrase a little about what the guest said and dig deeper into the comment with a follow-up question.

For example: "You mentioned that limited maternity leave support was a turning point in your career—can you walk us through how that experience shaped your approach to leadership?"

This process validates the speaker's emotions, invites elaboration, and creates an opportunity for the audience to reflect alongside the host. Even brief summarizing statements before moving on can help maintain continuity and build trust and rapport.

Dig deeper into a comment that was made by carrying a curious mindset. Rather than just being a host, this shows that you are actively seeking to learn just like the audience. However, if you are short on time and want to move onto the next question, comment briefly and think of a question related to the guest's response to show that you were listening, similar to a follow up question.

By applying these perspectives as a host, you are creating and crafting an interview that resonates with your audience's point of view. This approach is valuable in medical education podcasting, where nuanced clinical concepts need to be clearly communicated to healthcare professionals and students.

3. *Open-ended questions:*

It is essential to ask questions that give the speaker the freedom to elaborate and share meaningful insights. Open-ended questions are especially valuable, as they encourage expansive responses rather than simple "yes" or "no" answers. These types of questions allow guests to reflect, explain, and tell stories in their own words, which enhances the depth and quality of the conversation.

Open-ended questions typically begin with prompts such as:

- "Tell me about..."
- "How did you...?"
- "What was it like when...?"

These prompts invite storytelling and introspection, which are especially useful in educational and narrative-driven interviews.

What to Do If You Ask a Closed Question

Even experienced interviewers may occasionally ask a closed-ended question. When this happens, there are a few easy ways to recover:

1. **Follow up with an open-ended prompt:**
   Example: "Did you find that challenging?" → "What aspects of it were most difficult for you?"
2. **Use the phrase "In what ways...?"**
   Example: "Was it effective?" → "In what ways was it effective or not?"
3. **Ask for an example rather than a definition:**
   Example: "What do you mean by that?" ➔"Can you give an example of what that looked like in your experience?"

Additional Tips

- **Avoid multiple questions at once.** Multiple questions can confuse the guest and often result in only part of the question being answered.
- **Use closed questions sparingly.** While not ideal for most podcast interviews, closed-ended questions can be useful:
  - To clarify specific details (e.g., numbers, dates, yes/no facts).
  - To wrap up a topic before transitioning to a new subject.

4. *Using silence Strategically:*

Silence can be perceived as empty, awkward, or a sign of disapproval. As a result, podcast hosts may feel pressure to fill every pause with validating phrases like "mmhmm" or "okay," or to edit out silences during post-production. Commonly there is a focus on the mechanics of silence, as in counting seconds or pacing a conversation, rather than considering how to make the silence meaningful [8].

When used intentionally, silence is a powerful tool for connection. One of the most effective ways to create engaging, emotionally resonant interviews is by incorporating brief, purposeful pauses after a guest has finished speaking. These moments give listeners time to process the content and, just as importantly, allow guests the space to reflect. Often, the most revealing or vulnerable insights come after a moment of silence, when the guest thinks they've finished but chooses to go deeper [9].

Silence conveys presence. It signals that the host is not just waiting to speak but is truly listening. It has been reported that well-timed pauses in conversations signals that the listener is fully present and engaged with the speaker's emotional experience, making the speaker feel heard and understood [8]. This concept of "compassionate silence," particularly in pediatric clinical settings, has been shown to foster connection, trust, and emotional intimacy between clinicians, patients, and families [10]. Rather than rushing to respond, hosts can leave a few seconds of quiet, which often invites further elaboration or reflection. Awkward silences often happen when there's an unexpected pause in conversation, prompting someone to quickly fill the gap with something random or unintentional [10].

While verbal affirmations have their place, overusing them can disrupt the natural rhythm of the conversation. By embracing silence as an active, communicative element, podcast hosts can foster trust, invite vulnerability, and create a richer, more thoughtful listening experience. Here are examples of different scenarios of when to utilize silence strategically:

Examples of when to utilize silence strategically:

1. **After an emotional memory**
   When a guest shares something personal or difficult, a moment of silence can invite emotional vulnerability and signals them to continue, often leading to deeper reflection.

2. **Explaining complex concepts**
   If a guest uses overly technical language, staying quiet can prompt them to rephrase more accessibly without being directly asked.
3. **Reflecting on clinical errors or heavy experiences**
   When guests share emotionally charged clinical stories, a pause before responding shows respect and allows space to process.
4. **Audience-centered recap**
   When addressing listeners directly, silence becomes an instructional technique, giving the audience time to mentally engage before the answer is revealed.

Preparing Your Guests

Medical education podcasts often feature diverse experts to explore emerging issues, scientific papers, and new innovations in medicine [11]. Your guests are key players for providing unique knowledge and sparking curiosity and conversations in niche topics. By establishing clear expectations and formulating a plan beforehand, hosts can help their guests feel confident and ready to share their perspectives during the podcast recording. Whether providing questions in advance or maintaining a more spontaneous approach with broad topic outlines, proper preparation helps guests feel confident and ready to share their expertise effectively. This chapter explores strategies for guest preparation that lead to engaging, informative, and time-efficient podcast episodes. Here are important steps that will help prepare your invited guests on the podcast.

1. **Choosing the right guest:**

Thorough research and networking with other individuals can help you find an expert on the topic of choice. As a host, you must invest time in understanding your guest's professional background, reviewing their recent publications, learning about their clinical expertise and communication style. Read relevant scientific articles, guidelines, and recent developments in the field of your guest. Listen to other podcast appearances or recorded lectures to understand their communication and teaching style. By familiarizing yourself with their work and contributions to their field, you can ask insightful questions that will resonate with your audience and develop rapport with them. This research enables you to understand the field and craft a purposeful conversation that extracts meaningful insights. If you invite multiple guests, clarify each person's role to ensure the discussion highlights their distinct contributions.

2. **Set Clear Objectives and an Agenda:**

Before recording, it's important to create a clear and collaborative plan with your guest. Discuss the framework and expectations of the episode and work together to develop shared objectives. Brief your guests on your podcast including format, audience, and the recording process. You may want to outline the flow of the conversation or provide a written outline or interview questions to scaffold the conversation so that your guest knows what to expect [12]. This collaborative process should culminate in developing a central theme for listeners to takeaway.

Make sure to explain how the podcast works and address any technical questions they might have. While most medical education podcasts are audio-only, some incorporate visual elements such as images or video clips [13]. Based on your podcast's format, work with guests to determine if they would like to include any supplementary visual materials. Ensure that your guest is informed in advance about whether your podcast includes visual recordings.

3. **Interview structure**

The success of a podcast relies on maintaining a consistent structure that serves as a familiar framework to keep listeners engaged while also allowing them to anticipate the flow of each episode. For instance, the *KeyLIME Podcast: Key Literature in Medical Education* demonstrates the effectiveness of a defined format throughout over 250 episodes. Their episodes consistently follow a structured approach: beginning with discussions on medical literature, moving into methodological analysis, and concluding with a thorough evaluation of the article's strengths, weaknesses, and educational significance [11]. Inform guests of your podcast structure and the anticipated flow of the conversation.

To create a warm environment and establish rapport, the interview should begin with a welcoming introduction followed by highlighting the guest's expertise and achievements. To enhance the episode's authenticity, hosts can incorporate personal stories of their connection with the guest that will guide the conversation to create an intimate atmosphere. This opening segment helps establish credibility with the audience while creating a comfortable atmosphere for the conversation to take off. The conversation should then progress organically, with questions flowing naturally from foundational concepts to more sophisticated discussions.

4. **Time Management**

As a host, you should have a sense of how you want to manage time within an episode, while staying flexible to adapt to changes or guests who veer off topic. While it's helpful to have a structure, great conversations can't be micromanaged. If the guest offers unexpected insight, follow the thread—even if it means adjusting your plan. Let content, not the clock, drive the energy. Tips for hosts to manage timing and flow:

- **Set expectations for segment times:**
  - Introduction (2–3 min)
  - Main discussion (15–20 min)
  - Closing remarks (2–3 min).
- **Create natural transitions and pivot points:**
  - "That's a great point—and building on that…"
  - "Let's shift gears and talk about…"

- **Redirect gently when needed:**
  - "That's fascinating—maybe we can come back to that later, but I'd love to hear your thoughts on…"
  - "I want to be mindful of time, so let's move into…"
- **Thoughtfully edit:** Don't interrupt a thoughtful conversation unless necessary when extra material can be trimmed in post-editing. Stay present and let guests complete their thoughts.
- **Save the best for last:** Encourage guests to share key takeaways and self-promote at the end of the episode. Guests will want to save time for these important points.

Take a deep breath and enjoy the conversation. The best interviews are those that have genuine curiosity and casual conversations.

5. **Provide technical guidance**

It is very common for technical complications to occur at any time. Ensuring high production quality requires careful planning and clear communication between hosts and guests. A smooth recording experience depends on hosts providing all necessary technical requirements in advance, including details about the equipment needed for high-quality content. Hosts should not expect guests to have technical expertise in podcasting or equipment needs and should provide a jargon-free explanation in advance of the recording.

Audio quality significantly impacts podcast accessibility and acceptability across diverse listener populations. Hosts should not only use high-quality equipment themselves but also educate their guests on the benefits of using proper recording tools to enhance learning [14]. Key elements of a successful recording with high quality audio include:

- A quiet recording environment without background noise, echo, or reverberation
- Headphones to prevent audio feedback
- High-quality microphone

To facilitate a seamless setup, hosts should provide guests with download links for any necessary recording software and clear setup instructions. Providing detailed information about hardware and system requirements can help avoid technical issues that might arise during the recording process. Furthermore, ensuring a stable internet connection for remote recordings is crucial to prevent interruptions and maintain a consistent flow of conversation.

6. **Legalities of Medical education podcasts**

Legal considerations are fundamental to protecting your content and preventing potential lawsuits. Due to varying state laws regarding personal rights, particularly in states like California or Florida [15, 16], it's crucial to understand the legal implications of using someone's voice and personal information in a podcast. A proper release agreement should outline the terms of usage, including any compensation (monetary or non-monetary, such as publicity) or voluntary participation, and specify your rights to use their voice and shared information in the podcast. Create legal documents outlining the terms and conditions of your podcast. It has become more common practice for guests to provide consent either through a signed agreement via email or recorded verbal consent during the show [17]. Remind guests about maintaining patient privacy and HIPAA compliance. Podcasters have the duty to maintain transparency and integrity in their broadcast, which often includes disclosures.

7. **Post-interview**

Hosts should promptly express gratitude to all guests. Remember to communicate the release timeline of the episode, as it helps guests know when to expect the episode's publication and plan any promotional efforts. Additionally, providing guidelines for sharing the episode on their platforms can encourage guests to promote the episode, increasing its reach and engagement. By handling these post-recording steps efficiently, hosts can maximize the impact of each episode and maintain a professional relationship with their guests.

Improvisation Interview Skills

While medical interviews traditionally follow structured formats, incorporating elements of improvisation can provide more engaging and authentic conversations for the listener. Your ability to improvise allows for further exploration of insights that arise during the podcast. Successful use of improvisation in podcasts enables a more natural approach to exploring topics while maintaining the podcast's educational value for the listener.

Improvisational theater or improv is a performance technique built on spontaneity, active listening, and collaboration. Performers create scenes without a script, responding in real time to speakers or characters' words and actions. While traditionally rooted in the arts, improv has increasingly found relevance in medical training to better interact with patients, where its core principles are used to enhance communication, adaptability, and empathy [18]. In a pilot study, medical students found that improvisational exercises helped them connect more effectively with patients from diverse backgrounds by improving listening, observation, relationship-building, and adaptability [19]. Similarly, hosting a podcast often mirrors the dynamics of a live clinical interaction: engaging with another person, adapting to unexpected turns in conversation, and fostering trust through empathy and presence. The best podcast interviews are not back and forth question-and-answer sessions; they feel like real conversations.

By applying improv-based techniques, podcast hosts can feel more comfortable, build trust, and adapt to any conversation. Whether navigating a surprising guest comment or recovering from a momentary lapse, these skills help create compelling, human-centered dialogue. This section outlines key improv techniques that will elevate your interviews.

1. **Active listening:** Focus on being fully present and avoid thinking ahead to your next question, as this may make it difficult to employ improvisation strategies [20].

   - Allow for natural pauses
   - Ask clarifying questions or paraphrase important points to confirm understanding
   - Use non-verbal cues of engagement such as nodding

2. **Employ the "Yes, and…" Technique to Foster Collaborative Dialogue**
   At its core, "Yes, and…" means acknowledging the guest's comment, making them feel heard or validated. Next, follow up by adding your own insight, curiosity, or related experience [21, 22]. This method allows there to be point of connection in the conversation.

   This principle has increasingly been recognized for its impact on communication within clinical and educational environments. Clinicians who have adopted this technique have reported more productive discussions with patients and families, particularly with differing views on treatments and vaccinations [23]. This approach encourages active listening and helps build momentum in the conversation by affirming what was said and thoughtfully expanding on it.

   - "Yes, that's fascinating, and I'm curious about…"
   - "Yes, that's one perspective and another is…"

   This approach fosters collaboration, keeps energy flowing, and avoids the conversational roadblock of "No, but…", a phrase that can unintentionally shut down dialogue or come off as dismissive. While critical thinking and differing viewpoints are welcome, framing them constructively invites further discussion rather than derailing it.
3. **Flexibility:** Be willing to "follow the energy" of the conversation. In other words, it may be beneficial to pursue interesting tangents to the conversation that you believe may provide educational value. As a rule of thumb, if a guest becomes particularly animated or excited about a specific topic or aspect of their work, it can indicate that there is an opportunity to uncover unique insights.

   One way to continue the conversation is by using open-ended questions that facilitate elaboration on the topic.

   - If the guest is enthusiastic or animated: "You clearly love this work—what drew you to it initially?"

4. **Mirroring and reading nonverbal cues:** The mirroring technique involves imitating and reflecting the other person's body language, facial expressions, and movements to build rapport and trust [23]. Pay attention to your guest's body language and micro expressions, to monitor comfort level and interest in the topic of discussion. Are they nodding or showing other signs of engagement? Are they smiling, or are their eyes drifting away, indicating distraction or discomfort? This enables you to know when it is suitable to probe deeper into a certain topic of discussion or when it may be more appropriate to move on to a

Table 7.2 Non-verbal cues from a podcast guest

Non-verbal cues from a guest:	
Cues to Pursue the topic further	Cues to shift to a different topic:
Guest leans in further Maintains strong eye contact Offers detailed or elaborate responses Gestures enthusiastically while discussing a specific topic	Looks away frequently Reduces their eye contact Gives shorter or "clipped" answers Uses closed body language (crossed arms, hunched posture) Makes tense facial expression

different topic gracefully. Many non-verbal cues will not be available to you if recording in an audio-only format, but instead you can read tone, cadence, silence, and filler words (um's and ah's). Please see Table 7.2 to see further non-verbal cues from your podcast guest to monitor.

5. **Stay in the moment and have fun:** Before any interview, take a few moments to loosen up: stretch, do a vocal warm-up, or engage in a brief mindfulness exercise. Getting into the right mental state can help you feel more grounded and focused. It's completely normal to feel nervous, especially during high-stakes conversations. Simple techniques like deep breathing and staying hydrated can ease anxiety and sharpen your focus. Remember, podcasting, like improvisation, is meant to be dynamic and even a little playful. Mistakes will happen and this is normal, so don't dwell on them. Staying stuck in a moment of self-doubt can throw off your rhythm. Instead, keep moving forward with confidence.

   Effective improvisation in medical education podcast interviews requires a balance between preparation and spontaneity. Remember that this is a skill that takes time and practice to develop. Record practice interviews, seek feedback, and refine your approach based on feedback or responses from listeners and guests.

Conclusion

Mastering the role of a podcast host requires more than entertaining listeners or asking thought provoking questions. As this chapter has outlined, hosts are educators, technicians, and storytellers who bridge the gap between experts and listeners. From crafting narrative arcs and guiding emotionally resonant conversations to preparing guests, adapting in real-time, and fostering audience-centered communication, effective hosts create learning environments where complex ideas become accessible and memorable.

References

1. Kaplan H, Verma D, Sargsyan Z. What traditional lectures can learn from podcasts. J Grad Med Educ. 2020;12(3):250–3. https://doi.org/10.4300/jgme-d-19-00619.1.
2. Speer NK, Reynolds JR, Swallow KM, Zacks JM. Reading stories activates neural representations of visual and motor experiences. Psychol Sci. 2009;20(8):989–99. Epub 20090630. https://doi.org/10.1111/j.1467-9280.2009.02397.x. PubMed PMID: 19572969; PMCID: PMC2819196.
3. Riddell J, Robins L, Brown A, Sherbino J, Lin M, Ilgen JS. Independent and interwoven: a qualitative exploration of residents' experiences with educational podcasts. Acad Med. 2020;95(1):89–96. https://doi.org/10.1097/acm.0000000000002984. PubMed PMID: 31517682.
4. Stephens GJ, Silbert LJ, Hasson U. Speaker-listener neural coupling underlies successful communication. Proc Natl Acad Sci U S A. 2010;107(32):14425–30. Epub 20100726. https://doi.org/10.1073/pnas.1008662107. PubMed PMID: 20660768; PMCID: PMC2922522.
5. Murphy S, Melandri E, Bucci W. The effects of story-telling on emotional experience: an experimental paradigm. J Psycholinguist Res. 2021;50(1):117–42. Epub 20210208. https://doi.org/10.1007/s10936-021-09765-4. PubMed PMID: 33555538.
6. Downs JS. Prescriptive scientific narratives for communicating usable science. Proc Natl Acad Sci USA. 2014;111 Suppl 4(Suppl 4):13627–33. Epub 20140915. https://doi.org/10.1073/pnas.1317502111. PubMed PMID: 25225369; PMCID: PMC4183172.
7. Bosshard S, Rodero E, Rodríguez-de-Dios I, Brickner J. Radio, podcasts, and music streaming-an electroencephalography and physiological analysis of listeners' attitude, attention, memory, and engagement. Brain Sci. 2024;14(4). Epub 20240329. https://doi.org/10.3390/brainsci14040330. PubMed PMID: 38671982; PMCID: PMC11047838.
8. Kaye EC, Rockwell SL, Lemmon ME, Baker JN, Mack JW. The art of saying nothing. Pediatrics. 2022;149(6). https://doi.org/10.1542/peds.2022-056862. PubMed PMID: 35641466; PMCID: PMC9619411.
9. Bartels J, Rodenbach R, Ciesinski K, Gramling R, Fiscella K, Epstein R. Eloquent silences: a musical and lexical analysis of conversation between oncologists and their patients. Patient Educ Couns. 2016;99(10):1584–94. Epub 20160420. https://doi.org/10.1016/j.pec.2016.04.009. PubMed PMID: 27156659; PMCID: PMC6100772.
10. Back AL, Bauer-Wu SM, Rushton CH, Halifax J. Compassionate silence in the patient-clinician encounter: a contemplative approach. J Palliat Med. 2009;12(12):1113–7. https://doi.org/10.1089/jpm.2009.0175. PubMed PMID: 19698026; PMCID: PMC2939848.
11. Lomayesva NL, Martin AS, Dowley PA, Davies NW, Olyha SJ, Wijesekera TP. Five medical education podcasts you need to know. Yale J Biol Med. 2020;93(3):461–6. Epub 20200831. PubMed PMID: 32874153; PMCID: PMC7448387.
12. Miller KA, Keeney T, Fialkowski A, et al. Leveraging podcasts to introduce medical students to the broader community of health care professionals. MedEdPORTAL. 2021;17:11191. Epub 20211025. https://doi.org/10.15766/mep_2374-8265.11191. PubMed PMID: 34754938; PMCID: PMC8542682.
13. Kelly JM, Perseghin A, Dow AW, Trivedi SP, Rodman A, Berk J. Learning through listening: a scoping review of podcast use in medical education. Acad Med. 2022;97(7):1079–85. Epub 20220623. https://doi.org/10.1097/acm.0000000000004565. PubMed PMID: 34935729; PMCID: PMC11002568.
14. Brust T, Yeung M. Clinical neuroscience podcasts for family medicine, internal medicine, and neurology residents: a needs assessment study (P1. 312). Neurology. 2014;82(10_supplement):P1. 312.
15. Library CS. Copyright Policy - California State Library. 2021. Available from: https://www.library.ca.gov/california-history/fair-use/.

16. State FDo. Copyright | Terms of use n.d. Available from: https://dos.fl.gov/copyright/.
17. Merlin. The legal side of podcasting: what you need to know. Wavve; 2024. Available from: https://wavve.co/the-legal-side-of-podcasting-what-you-need-to-know/.
18. Neel N, Maury JM, Heskett KM, Iglewicz A, Lander L. The impact of a medical improv curriculum on wellbeing and professional development among pre-clinical medical students. Med Educ Online. 2021;26(1):1961565. https://doi.org/10.1080/10872981.2021.1961565. PubMed PMID: 34412576; PMCID: PMC8381956.
19. Rusiecki JM, Orlov NM, Dolan JA, Smith MP, Zhu M, Chin MH. Exploring the value of improvisational theater in medical education for advancing the doctor-patient relationship and health equity. Acad Med. 2023;98(6s):S46–s53. Epub 20230523. https://doi.org/10.1097/acm.0000000000005183. PubMed PMID: 36811964; PMCID: PMC10286128.
20. Fu B. Common ground: frameworks for teaching improvisational ability in medical education. Teach Learn Med. 2019;31(3):342–55. Epub 20181231. https://doi.org/10.1080/10401334.2018.1537880. PubMed PMID: 30596300.
21. Weger JH, R. CG, Emmett MC. Active listening in peer interviews: the influence of message paraphrasing on perceptions of listening skill. Int J Listen. 2010;24(1):34–49. https://doi.org/10.1080/10904010903466311.
22. Gunderman RB. Education in professionalism: improvisation. Acad Radiol. 2016;23(5):655–7. Epub 20160302. https://doi.org/10.1016/j.acra.2015.12.022. PubMed PMID: 26947222.
23. Mehta A, Fu B, Chou E, Mitchell S, Fessell D. Improv: transforming physicians and medicine. Med Sci Educ. 2021;31(1):263–6. Epub 20201201. https://doi.org/10.1007/s40670-020-01174-x. PubMed PMID: 34457880; PMCID: PMC8368394.

Chapter 8
Post-production Skills

Doug Nagel

What Is Post-production?

Post-production. That's a broad term that seems to apply to *everything* after "production." Where is this imaginary line drawn that separates the production from post-production? Once you've gotten that fantastic recording from your hosts and guests, and they've committed all those delicious nuggets of information onto tape (or, rather, a file), there is still much work to be done to make it into the show that will delight and educate your listeners and be consumed by countless fans. That's where post-production comes in, and it happens once the audio recording is done. Post-production for a podcast is taking all of the raw audio recordings and transforming them into a final, polished show that is ready for the world. This includes cleaning up the audio, editing the show, adding music and sound effects, structuring the episode, and exporting the show in the proper format.

Go Team! (or Maybe Just Go You)

There are several roles that participate in producing a regular podcast. I say roles and not team members, because many of these can overlap and might be the same person. Depending on the size of the production, they might *all* be one person. That can be a lot of hats to wear! Let's look at these roles and see who's who—and who's you.

D. Nagel (✉)
American Academy of Pediatrics, Itasca, IL, USA
e-mail: dnagel@aap.org

J. Parga-Belinkie et al. (eds.), *Podcasting for Medical Professionals*,
https://doi.org/10.1007/978-3-032-16480-3_8

The front face (or voice) of the podcast is the host. This is the person with the golden voice that is conducting the interview. This person is the chief representative and the image of your show. A charismatic and captivating host will draw listeners in by developing an "on air" personality that keeps listeners engaged from show to show and makes them feel like they are part of something bigger. They become a community or a family with the host and that bond grows stronger every time they listen. The host may also contribute in other ways by writing scripts, recommending guests, and suggesting topics. Hosts will also be instrumental in marketing for the show, appearing in materials, graphics and promotions. People like to put a face to the voice, even if the actual podcast is an audio-only show.

The producer is a major part of the podcast and generally holds and pulls it all together. Producers typically decide what direction the show is going in and guide it along. They book guests, write scripts, and make content decisions. The producer is in on the recording of the show and is listening for content, guiding the hosts and guests and shaping the show. When they are guiding, this doesn't mean they are micromanaging the recording. A good producer can be hands-on without being overbearing. As a producer, you are also a director. You have to know when to step in and help coach and guide for a great bite and when to fade into the background and let the hosts and guests just talk if they are in a rhythm. It is the producer's job to help them find that rhythm. The producer makes sure their hosts are ready and makes guests feel comfortable and confident enough to give their best during the recording. A good producer can help a first-time guest feel like a veteran by the end of their first recording, and they will want to be back on again in the future!

While the producer focuses mostly on the creative side of the show, the executive producer is more focused on the business side of things. The executive producer manages things at the top level. They are usually the money folks, procuring funds for the show and managing how and where those funds are spent. They make sure that operations are on time and within budget. Executive producers will also make sure that the show consistently aligns with its mission and vision. Both the producer and executive producer overlap and align on some of these aspects.

The producer also overlaps with the editor, and many times they are the same person. The editor takes the rough show and shapes it into what will become the final product, trimming the fat and keeping the good stuff. They are in the transcript deleting pieces and moving sections. They are in the audio software cutting the show. The editor is responsible for making the producer's vision a reality—the best version of that reality it can be. That's why they are often the same person or will work very closely together.

The audio engineer is responsible for making everyone sound their best. During the recording, the audio engineer is the one pressing record. They could be running the session if everyone is in a studio recording together, making sure everyone is dialed in and sounding great. Over a remote session, the engineer may be listening for irregular sounds and noises on everyone's tracks as they record or providing assistance for optimum setup. The audio engineer is listening to the technical side of things so the producer can focus on the content. Table 8.1 below is a summary of the roles discussed above.

Table 8.1 The different hats that you and/or your team will wear

Job	Description
Host	The voice (and face) of the show, conducts the interviews
Producer	Guides the show, directs, books guests, writes scripts, makes content decisions
Executive producer	Manages all aspects at the top level, procures money, keeps operations on time and in budget
Editor	Cuts show into polished product
Audio engineer	Run recording session, make everyone sound their best

Editing (and Some Important Things That Go with It)

You've probably heard the phrase tossed around from time to time, "We'll fix it in post," meaning let's get all of this stuff recorded and we'll worry about problems later. That guest was great, but some of their answers maybe veered off-topic or went on for a bit too long. Perhaps they were a remote guest on the show and maybe their home or office audio setup was not quite up to snuff. Not everyone has a professional-grade microphone and sound booth just hanging around in their home or office! This is where you will perform some necessary editing to begin to shape the show into a final product. If you are wearing the editor or engineer hat on your team, fixing it in post will, most likely, fall to you.

Let me begin by stating, first off, that "fixing it in post" is not always the way you will want to do things. If you can fix an issue when it's happening (or before it even happens), that's even better. It can be the difference between a smooth edit and a nightmare. If you're not recording all of your episodes in a fancy podcast studio where the guests and the hosts all have the same setup in the same room, there will be more variables to consider that will affect your show. Maybe your guests are remote, calling in from their home or office for the recording. You can find out a lot about what your remote guest is going to sound like by having a rehearsal meeting first. That will give you a chance to see what they are working with, listen to how they sound, and make recommendations on how they can get the best sound with what they have. If they have nothing (or none of it sounds particularly good), this can also give you a chance to make some quick equipment recommendations that will benefit them (and you) every time they are a guest on the show. What they use to record, the room they are in, the microphone they are using, and the way they are using it can all play a part in what they are going to sound like. Doing a little "pre-editing" can really go a long way to helping your edit be more manageable.

Part of the post-production process that happens around the edit (I personally like to do it beforehand) is audio engineering. As we go forward and discuss the editing process, we are going to make the assumption that everything is being recorded digitally to files and being edited via computer. There are other ways to do this, but this is certainly the most common and efficient. You'll first want to take your individual voices and line them up within what's called a multitrack. A multitrack is really a timeline where all the different voices can play back all at once, and the editing software you choose should be able to do that. Each voice will be on its own discrete track so each can be individually "sweetened" to your liking.

Although having discrete tracks is ideal and preferred, it's not always possible depending on what's available. There are instances where people might be using meeting software, such as Zoom or Teams, to make their recordings. This will put the audio all on one track. You might be thinking, "Great! That's less to keep track of." While that may be true, the files that come from these programs are often produced in what are called compressed and lossy formats. Compressed, in this context, means that the file has been condensed into a smaller size than it would otherwise be. This compressing of the file results in "lossy" audio. This means that information and portions of the audio spectrum are missing. Think of when you speak to someone on the phone. While the tech has vastly improved over time, a phone call does not sound the same as being in-person. There is sonic information missing from what you are hearing. That's not to say don't use these programs to record. If this is what's available, record and get the show!

Start by taking a quick listen to everyone individually and get acquainted with everyone's voice. How does everyone sound? If you got excellent sound from your hosts and guests during the recording, then great! That makes this part simpler. You'll want to listen for noise on the individual tracks. This can be made even easier by making sure to record 10–15 seconds of "room tone," or silence with no one talking, during the recording. Does anyone have any hissing or excessive room noise going on? Maybe the heat or air conditioning was running and the mic picked it up. Maybe the track contains a consistent hum or buzz from a power source or a computer fan. These sorts of things almost always make it through to the recording in some way, even when being extra careful during the recording. This unwanted stuff in the background of your otherwise pristine recording is called the noise floor. When recording, you want maximum voice with a low noise floor. The most common background noises you might hear can often be remedied with a noise reduction program. Many of the editing programs available (free or not) will have noise reduction software built in or available for purchase. Two great examples of free (and also popular) software with full feature sets are Audacity, and Apple's own GarageBand. Every Mac, iPhone and iPad comes with GarageBand installed, and Audacity is available online for a free download. I am a fan of noise reduction because any other processing that you do to any track that involves raising the volume of the speaker will also raise the noise floor. The lower the noise floor is, the better and clearer your speaker will be heard. This is also why you want to check for noise and fix it first, before you do anything else to a track.

Now that the tracks are clean, it's time to make them sound their best. We are not going to get too deep in the weeds here on audio processing and techniques—that's a whole other book in and of itself! I would encourage you to do a deeper dive on some of the terms and processes mentioned herein to gain a greater understanding of what they do and precisely how they work. As you work more with different voices, you'll be able to tell what they need just from your initial listen.

The first thing we are listening for is dynamics or dynamic range. Dynamic range is the volume of the voice throughout the recording as it was recorded, from the lowest tones to the highest peaks. This is also a visual process, because you can see the waveforms in your editing software from start to finish. Unless you're going for a specific effect, you'll want those dynamics to be consistent throughout the track. You could go through the entire track and attempt to raise and lower the volume at all of the spots you want, but that would prove to be a very tedious and time-consuming exercise. The best way to control and tame dynamics is to use what's called a compressor. A compressor, at its most basic, does right by its namesake. It compresses signals to help to even out the dynamics. Please see Fig. 8.1 below for a pictural description.

This is different than the compression we discussed earlier for files. This kind of compression is the good stuff when it's used correctly! There are hundreds of compressors available in hardware and software, and pretty much every piece of editing software includes at least one in its arsenal. Some of them will have an array of controls, others may condense controls down to one knob or slider. A compressor can be difficult to understand, Fig. 8.2 takes us through the operation as the signal passes through it. Imagine that the signal passes through in a straight line, and each step of the compressor's process is a point on that line.

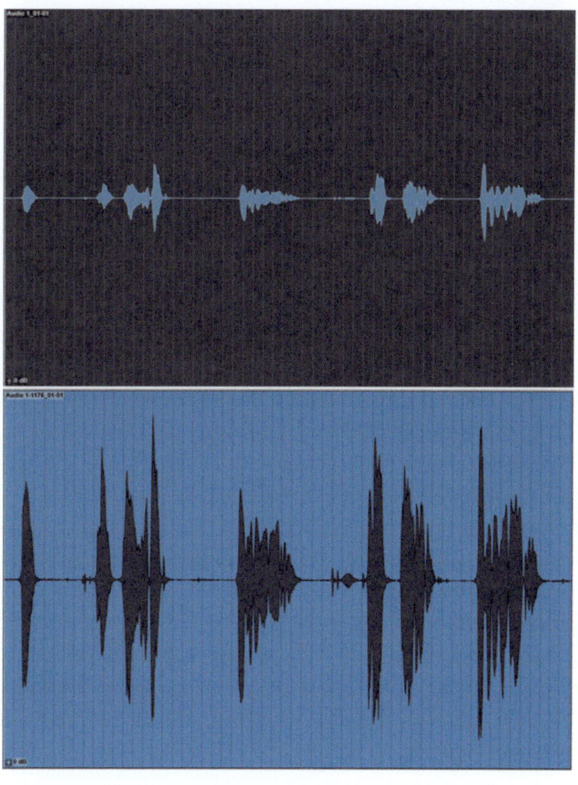

Fig. 8.1 A line of spoken dialog. The top is the raw signal, and the bottom is the compressed one

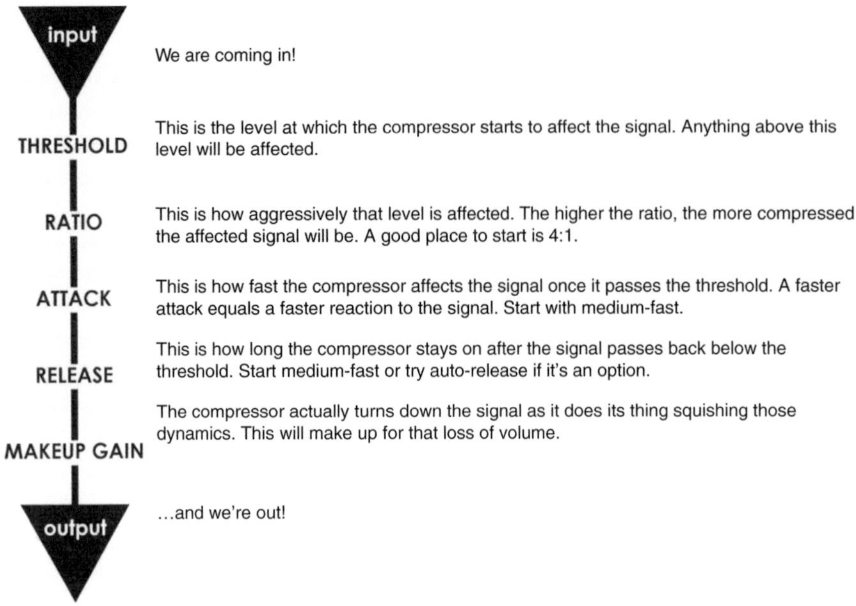

Fig. 8.2 A chart explaining audio traveling through the steps of a compressor

As I said before, not all compressors will have all these controls, but this process is what they are all doing inside. Most importantly, while doing this process, listen. These processes often don't require extreme measures for good results. Listen and know that it's right if it sounds right!

A compressor can be your best friend if you are working with a single track instead of discrete tracks. Let's say you get your recording from Zoom or Teams and one person is obviously louder than the others. You can't exactly turn down their track because it's all baked into one file. You can, however, send this track through a compressor to even everyone out. The compressor will smooth out the dynamics, bringing up the lower voices and tamping down the loud ones, and now everyone is on the same level!

After fixing the dynamics, I will usually go to equalization, or EQ, next, if it's deemed necessary. EQ-ing a signal is the raising or lowering of certain frequencies across the spectrum (measured in Hertz, Hz) to shape a sound. Figure 8.3 shows is the frequency range of human hearing for reference. Generally, I apply the "less is more" concept when I do this process. I tend to carve out, or remove, problem frequencies by subtracting rather than adding all around them. EQ can be thought of as a line as well, and it's often represented that way, ranging from low to high frequencies.

As you experiment with adding or removing frequencies across the spectrum, you'll find that some are more pleasing or helpful than others, and some ranges are entirely unnecessary. For example, you'll find that nothing really useful happens with your guests' voices below 70–80 Hz, so you can roll that off, eliminating low noise and rumble. How or if you use an EQ will also depend on the environment the voice was recorded in. Every room sounds different and has its own characteristics. What you'll want to do is use the EQ to tame unwanted frequencies that seem to "stick out" or add where there are deficiencies. This is a tool that should be used conservatively, listening to the changes as you go. As you practice using it, you'll find that you know what a voice needs (or doesn't) just by listening. This is a visual and aural process, and the visual part can make it easier to implement. Most programs will come with a spectrum analyzer or frequency analyzer. If you turn this tool on, you'll be able to see those frequencies hitting across the spectrum in real time. I use this tool every time to help me and my ears confirm what I need to remove and what I can add.

The next tool I like to use, if it's necessary, is what's called a de-esser. Some people you record may have very pronounced or exaggerated "esses," and you can use this tool to fix just that! Again, most editing software will have this built into it somewhere. The de-esser is actually another form of compressor, but it just focuses on a certain, defined frequency range. This is another process where you can use both your ears and eyes to get the best results. Your ears will definitely let you know there's a troubling "ess" in there, and your eyes can help to confirm where in the frequency range it's located. Set the de-esser to the frequency range where the offending "ess" is and use the threshold (sound familiar?) to tame it. The deeper the threshold, the more it will push down that "ess."

There's a reason why I've mentioned these things in this particular order. This is generally the order that you'll want to do these processes, because each one affects the next one. Noise reduction comes first. Then, unless I'm going for a specific sound, I adjust the dynamics before the EQ, so I am adding the EQ on top of my dynamically adjusted voice instead of smushing it. I apply the de-esser after the EQ because I can add high frequencies to make things a bit crispier on the top end (very technical term) and still tame those "esses." If I changed the order, I'm likely to bring those "esses" out even more. But…there may be times when you will need to change the order up a bit. If you have a very troubling frequency in the voice or a really extreme "ess" sound right off the bat, you might consider one of these processes before the dynamics, because the exaggeration, when left in, will change the way the voice hits the compressor. You might use an EQ to pull out an offending tone before dynamics and another one after to make your refinements. See Fig. 8.4 below for a pictural summary of what we're discussing. You can always try and experiment with this, because these rules are meant to be bent. No matter how you get your end product, it's good if it sounds good!

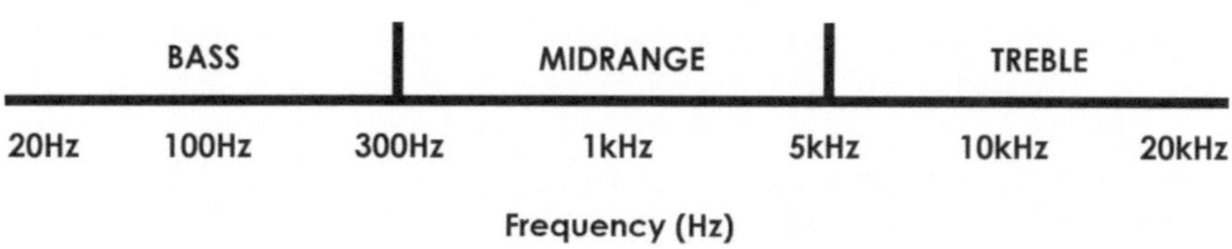

Fig. 8.3 Frequency range of human hearing from 20 Hz to 20 kHz

Now that our talent sounds great, we're going to switch hats and put on the editor's cap. We will take our individual voices and process them together into one track, often called a mixdown. Most editing software will have a mixdown function, where the software combines all of the tracks together and spits out one master file. This is the file we will edit. Before just going in and chopping up the audio, it can be very helpful to do what's called a paper edit. A paper edit is like a roadmap for your audio edit. You're taking the transcript of the show and making cuts within the transcript, crossing out pieces that you feel need to be cut and/or moving pieces around to get the best show you can. There are online services as well as software programs that will take your file, "listen" to it, and provide you with a timecoded transcript you can edit right on your computer. No actual paper needed!

While making these cuts, are you going in with a scalpel and being precise, or are you charging in with a chainsaw and cutting large swaths of programming out? Either method, or both, may be appropriate depending on the material. When making these decisions as you listen and read through your program, how long does your show need to be? Trimming a few words here and there for clarity will be the scalpel. Are there answers that run on for a long time and don't get to the meat of the matter right away? Get out the chainsaw. There are no hard and fast rules for total length but consider your end product and your audience when deciding. Put yourself in the listener's shoes and listen objectively. Consider how people consume podcasts (or how you consume them). Many folks listen on a commute or when they travel. They might listen during a workout or a lunch break. You want your content to be entertaining, interesting, well-informed and fit into these listening opportunities.

With your completed paper edit roadmap, you're ready to do the audio edit. I keep these pieces side-by-side on my screens and follow the transcript while

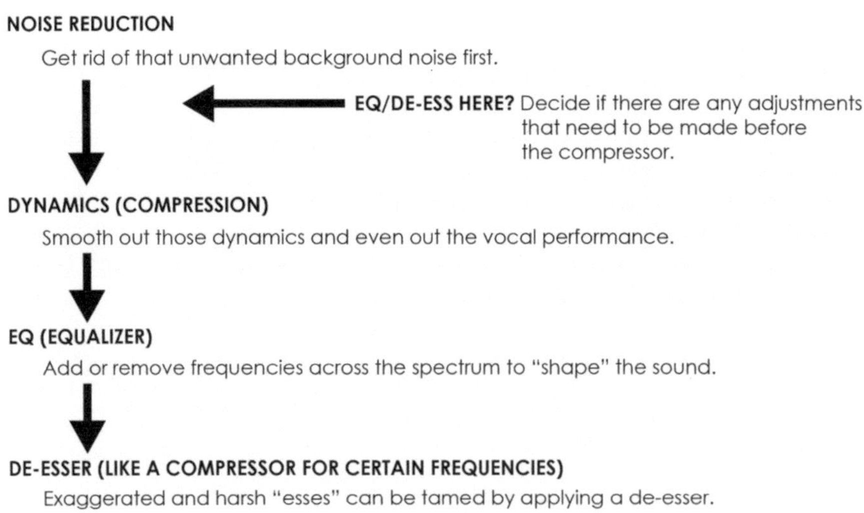

Fig. 8.4 The order of things. Don't forget to experiment!

listening to the audio. You want your guests and hosts to sound their best, but also natural and realistic. Are there big pauses where someone is looking for the right words? Cut those down to tighten up the show. If someone is heavy on the "umms," I like to cut those out. I personally will cut nearly all of them out unless an "umm" is part of another essential word and it sounds strange when I remove it. Some speakers will make a SMACK sound with their mouths when taking a breath or starting a phrase. These are annoying to me as an editor and a listener, so I will always try to remove or minimize them. Some people are "umm smackers" and will do both as a filler as they form their answers. Those are definitely getting removed from my show! As you are cutting pieces out of your mixdown, most software editing programs will do what's called a ripple edit, meaning that the audio track will close up the gaps as you cut pieces out and move the rest of the track up. The editing process is about how the show feels as well as how it sounds. Listen as you make these cuts. Does the cadence still sound natural? You don't want to have your interview sound like it was cut to pieces, even if it was. Make sure while you are cutting that there are no cut-off breaths or words left behind. It's unprofessional, and they will be noticed by your listeners and distract them. Always listen back to the edits as you are making them. Utilize the tools at your disposal. If you accidentally cut something out or chop a word in half, the undo command is your friend! Sometimes a carefully placed fade at the beginning or end of an edit, be it a breath or word, can make the difference and cover your tracks. Most editing software will allow you to do that along with straight cutting. Make sure your edits sound smooth. If they don't sound right to you, chances are someone else will notice.

Are you short on time? There are even software tools that will do all the work for you! Sites like Auphonic will utilize AI algorithms to do the work of an engineer and editor by cleaning up and balancing your tracks. While this may be an option (or *the* option) for some, I prefer to do these processes myself. I have been an audio engineer for nearly 30 years, and I enjoy the work and prefer to make those decisions myself. AI can be a great helper, but it will decide what it thinks is best, not necessarily what *you* think is best.

Peer Review (Get by with a Little Help from Your Friends)

You've got your show edited, and you think it's pretty great. Why wouldn't it be? You've dotted the I's and crossed the T's, trimmed the excess and kept the best nuggets. Before it goes out into the wild, it wouldn't be a bad idea to have a trusted source give it a review. Sometimes, it can be good to get a review from more than one source, just to make sure there is some objectivity in the process. When you edit and produce something, it can be hard to take yourself out of it and approach it objectively. Those hats you wore through the process, however many it was, tend to stay on even after it's done.

There are a couple important considerations you'll want in a peer review for your podcast. The first is someone who can listen to the material to make sure it is sound and accurate and that there are no holes in it. You may feel that you know the subject backwards and forwards, but material can go missing or get lost during the process. A reviewer listening to the content closely that is well-versed in the subject will be able to confirm that all is well.

You'll also want to know how it *sounds.* Having someone with a good ear can be very helpful to make sure that your edits are good and tight, without any cut-off breaths or words. They can listen to the pacing and confirm that the show *feels* right. They can also confirm that everything is as good as it can be sonically. Sometimes a second set of ears will pick up on something that you might have missed.

Peer review can also happen at other stages of the process. It might not be a bad idea to insert a review *before* making the edit. Once you have your paper edit, you could share it with your executive producer to make sure that the show is headed in the right direction. They may have insights into the subject matter and how it will be received by the listening public—more big picture observations.

Promotion and Marketing (If You Build It, Will They Come?)

The show is ready for the world…but how will the world know? You need to expand your audience by getting more exposure for the show. You'll get that exposure through promotion and marketing. You'll also be able to recoup your budget. This is one of those instances where you may need to spend money to make money. If you have some of your budget allotted for promotion and marketing, the return will (hopefully) allow you to increase your budget and continue production. If your budget is near zero to begin with, there are cheap and/or free options to find listeners as well.

Let's look at free first. Social media can be a great partner for your show. Most social media accounts are free and so is posting on them. Consider posting in feeds and groups of like-minded people, such as Facebook or LinkedIn pages specifically for pediatricians. You can promote your show within your network of social contacts by posting links to new episodes on your feeds—nothing wrong with tooting your own horn a little! The hope is that your fellow social contacts will see your posts and discover your show, sharing it along the way. When they see it and share, their friends see it and share, and you've got organic growth!

Another option that will cost you time but not necessarily money is sponsorship. You'll have to be a bit of a salesperson for this one, but you might be able to find a brand or organization that supports and believes in your vision and is willing to buy ad time on your show. If your show does well enough, they may even come looking for you! Podcast hosting services will often have spots for you to insert a pre-roll or a mid-roll (beginning or middle) ad in your show. If you can get a sponsor (or two) this can go a long way to paying the show's bills.

If you know anyone with a show that is already a success, you might be able to convince them to do a show with you to gain exposure. You could potentially gain listeners from their audience quickly, because they have an established on-air family/community. There's nothing wrong with a little cross-promotion, and both of your audiences and shows can benefit.

As we get into paid territory, we start again with social media and online ads. In addition to all the free posting you can do; you can also purchase ads that will show up on other people's feeds with similar interests. This is a great way to get a lot of notice quickly. You can also invest in a platform such as Google ads, which will allow you to spend a set amount of money on your ad campaign per month, per day, or even by the click. Once you've spent the allotted money, the ad will stop running until you add more.

You could buy ad time to play on other platforms that carry podcasts (like Spotify, for example) or even broadcast or satellite radio. This will get you some exposure for sure, but it is also a considerable monetary investment. Also, you'll need to record an ad! You would most likely have your host voice the ad and you would produce it with your team, so you would save on those costs at the very least.

Conclusion

Now we have reviewed all the different roles associated with a podcast and all the steps required to take a raw audio clip and turn it into a finished podcast ready to be released. We hope this chapter demystified post production skills and you enjoy creating your podcast.

Chapter 9
Marketing Your Medical Education Podcast

David Hill

Content First: Make It Great Before You Market

Before you focus on your marketing strategy, make sure you've absorbed and integrated the advice in this book's other chapters and developed a podcast people want to hear. Any marketing professional will tell you they can help your product gain exposure, but they can't work miracles. If you have a compelling product, your listeners will spread the word. Devoted listeners beat any marketing strategy you can come up with. Likewise, if your podcast doesn't engage its audience in the first minute (yes, those first 60 seconds), there's little even the best marketing strategy can do to help you gain a foothold in the market. In a world where attention is arguably the most valuable commodity, listeners demand you earn the moments they give you.

Finding Your Audience

Now that you have a superb product, how do you grow your audience? When potential learners are scrolling across multiple options, do your graphics stand out as bold and professional? Does your title tell them exactly what they're going to get and, importantly, match the tone of your production? Do the first notes of your musical introduction set a tone (literally) for what's to follow? A strong front-end investment in these stylistic components will help ensure listeners find the substance behind them. The goal is to create a podcast that not only delivers

D. Hill (✉)
University of Washington/Seattle Children's Hospital, Seattle, WA, USA

J. Parga-Belinkie et al. (eds.), *Podcasting for Medical Professionals*,
https://doi.org/10.1007/978-3-032-16480-3_9

high-quality medical education but also attracts and retains a dedicated audience. This involves careful planning and execution in several key areas, from visual branding to content promotion.

Choosing a Podcast Title: Clarity and Discoverability

This podcast is your baby, so you'll have to give it a name. The title of your podcast is often the first thing potential listeners will see, so it needs to be both informative and intriguing. As part of your research, you should have already assessed competitors in your market, so hopefully you have a list of names that are already taken. With this step out of the way, it may help you to envision your ideal listener. Where are they coming from? What would pique their interest? Check out the tips below and then jot down a list of words that come to mind in a column.

Now think about how you're positioning your podcast. Is it funny? Serious? Conversational? Academic? Is it based on a particular host's personality, or is the host more in service to the message? Make another list of words that answer these questions in a second column. Now start making connections between the two lists. Ideally come up with at least five different possible titles, then run them past members of your target audience. They should tell you quickly which title they'd click on and which they'd scroll right past. A focus group, even an informal one, can provide invaluable insights into how your target audience perceives your potential titles.

Key factors to consider when selecting:

- **Relevance:** Does the title clearly communicate your podcast's subject?
- **SEO Optimization:** Does it include keywords that medical professionals might search for?
- **Memorability:** Is it easy to say, spell, and remember?
- **Branding Consistency:** Does it align with your overall theme and messaging?

Consider incorporating keywords that your target audience is likely to search for. For example, if your podcast focuses on cardiology, including the word "cardiology" in the title can improve its visibility in search results. However, avoid keyword stuffing, as this can make your title sound unnatural and less appealing. Aim for a balance between clarity and searchability. Also, check if the name is available as a domain name and social media handle to ensure branding consistency across all platforms.

Examples of Effective Podcast Titles:

- **[Specialty] Update:** (e.g., "The Cardiology Update")—Simple, direct, and clearly communicates the subject matter
- **[Host Name] on [Medical Topic]:** (e.g., "Dr. Smith on Diabetes")—Personalizes the podcast and highlights the host's expertise
- **The [Adjective] Guide to [Medical Topic]:** (e.g., "The Essential Guide to Emergency Medicine")—Promises comprehensive coverage of a specific topic

Graphics: Establishing a Strong Visual Identity

Looks aren't everything, but no one can deny they draw your attention. We may not judge a book by its cover, but if the cover doesn't speak to us, we're a lot less likely to flip through the pages. In the crowded podcasting landscape, visual appeal is paramount. Your podcast's "cover" will appear as a little box on a screen among a bunch of other little boxes, so how will listeners know that yours is the one that holds the treasure they seek? The cover art should be striking yet simple, immediately communicating the subject matter and target audience. A well-designed cover can be the difference between a potential listener scrolling past your podcast and clicking to learn more.

Best practices for podcast cover design include:

- A **clean and uncluttered layout** with bold, readable fonts
- A **color scheme** that aligns with medical or educational branding (e.g., shades of blue, green, and white, which evoke trust and professionalism)
- A **strong, recognizable logo** that can be used across different media (e.g., website, merchandise, social media)

Consider the psychology of color when selecting your palette. Blue often conveys trust and stability, while green can suggest growth and health. White provides a sense of cleanliness and clarity, all essential in the medical field. Ensure that your logo is versatile and scalable, maintaining its clarity whether it's displayed on a small podcast app icon or a large banner at a medical conference. Also, think about creating a style guide that outlines the specific fonts, colors, and imagery to use across all your branding materials. This will help maintain a consistent and professional look.

You may have a design background or have a friend or family member who is skilled in the visual arts. If so, then you might turn to a professional design tool like Canva, Adobe Express, or Affinity Designer to help you create polished artwork. These tools offer a range of templates and features that can simplify the design process.

If not, however, it may be well worth your time to invest in the services of a design professional. Don't know anyone? No problem! Hiring a designer via personal connections or via an online marketplace ensures a professional touch. Be sure to evaluate a sample of their prior work and make sure they have the skills to portray your podcast's tone in a visual medium. Look for designers with experience in creating branding for healthcare or education, as they will be more familiar with the visual language that resonates with your target audience.

Additional Tips for Graphics:

- **Consistency:** Maintain a consistent visual style across all your podcast artwork, including cover art, social media graphics, and website visuals

- **Accessibility:** Ensure your graphics are accessible to individuals with visual impairments by using alt text for images and choosing color combinations with sufficient contrast
- **Updates:** Periodically refresh your cover art to keep it looking modern and relevant but avoid making drastic changes that could confuse your audience

Selecting Music: Setting the Right Tone

Do you ever close your eyes or look away from the screen during a movie or television show? What do you hear, and how does it affect your mood? Sometimes we focus so much on the visual that we miss how much the music and sound contribute to our experience of entertainment. In the realm of medical education podcasts, music plays a vital role in setting the tone and creating a cohesive listening experience.

A podcast may come with visuals, but most of your audience will experience it as a purely auditory format. As such, the opening beats of your cast will set a mood that is bound to influence their experience. Think about the atmosphere you want to create. Do you want listeners to feel relaxed and engaged, or energized and motivated? The right music can help you achieve this. One way to proceed is to go back to your lists from the above exercise and think about what sound projects your vision for this product.

Here again you may have relevant experience. Perhaps you studied music composition and performance, and you can sit down with a music recording program and create exactly the sound you're looking for. If you're like most people, however, you're going to need some help. Fortunately, there are more options than ever available to you, and they're not all expensive.

Consider:

- **Licensing:** Use royalty-free music from platforms to avoid copyright issues
- **Consistency:** Stick with a recognizable intro and outro to build familiarity
- **Mood Appropriateness:** The tone should reflect the professionalism of medical education—avoid overly dramatic or casual tunes

When selecting music, consider the tempo, instrumentation, and overall feel. A slower tempo can create a sense of calm and focus, while a faster tempo can convey energy and excitement. Instrumentation can also play a role; for example, acoustic instruments may sound more natural and approachable, while electronic instruments can create a more modern and technological feel. It is crucial to ensure that the music does not distract from the content. The music should complement the spoken word, not compete with it.

Additional Tips for Music Selection:

- **Brevity:** Keep your intro and outro music concise, ideally under 15 to 20 seconds
- **Volume:** Ensure the music is at a consistent volume level throughout the podcast and does not overpower the host's voice

- **Transitions:** Use smooth transitions between the music and spoken word to create a seamless listening experience

Crafting a professional and cohesive brand identity through graphics, title, and music will help your podcast stand out and not only reach but retain your target audience. These elements work together to create a memorable and engaging experience for listeners, ultimately contributing to the success of your medical education podcast.

Advertisers and Funding

Whether you're embarking on this journey as a public service or as an entrepreneur hoping to build a profitable side gig, you cannot avoid financial considerations. The costs associated with producing a high-quality medical education podcast can add up quickly, so it's important to have a clear understanding of your financial resources and potential revenue streams. Direct costs include equipment, hosting, editing, and marketing. High-quality microphones, editing software, and hosting platforms can be expensive, and professional editing services can further increase your costs.

Then there's the value of your time. What would you bring in if you spent this time moonlighting or consulting, for example? How do you value your time with family, friends, pursuing other hobbies? Before starting a podcast, you'll want to have a number in your head and then revisit it periodically to ensure that this project remains the best possible use of your energy. Consider not only the time spent recording and editing but also the time spent researching topics, preparing scripts, and promoting your podcast.

This podcast may be a passion project for you or an investment you're willing to make. In either case, you'll want to draw up a realistic business plan that accounts for all the likely costs and consider whether the expense is worth the personal or financial return you hope to gain. A well-structured business plan can help you identify potential funding sources, track expenses, and measure the success of your podcast.

If you're partnering with an institution like your hospital or professional society for this podcast, are your values aligned with theirs? It's essential to have a clear understanding of each party's expectations and responsibilities to avoid conflicts down the road. What happens when you want to cover a topic or interview a guest they find uncomfortable or risky? What degree of editorial control do they expect, what do you expect, and does your contract clearly state who has final say? A written agreement can protect both parties and ensure that the podcast remains true to its mission. Will you need sign-off for each episode, and if so, how long will that take and who will have the power to clear it for air?

If you're planning to fund your project through private sponsors or advertisers, how do you feel about relaying their message in your voice or under your imprimatur? Maintaining your credibility is paramount, so it's crucial to carefully consider the ethical implications of accepting sponsorships from certain companies. Perhaps you're fine touting the advantages of a particular mattress or insurance company, but what about pharmaceuticals, dietary supplements or "wellness" therapies? It's essential to have a clear ethical framework in place to guide your decisions about which sponsors to partner with. If you're lucky enough to reach a wide audience with medical information, advertisers will be eager to reach your listeners, too, and you'll want to think hard in advance about what you consider ethical.

Below are some models for funding your podcast.

Sponsorships: Partnering with Relevant Advertisers

Sponsorships can provide a steady stream of revenue for your podcast, but it's essential to choose sponsors that align with your values and target audience.

Potential sponsors include:

- **Pharmaceutical companies** looking to reach healthcare professionals
- **Medical device manufacturers** promoting new innovations
- **Medical associations and societies** interested in supporting professional education
- **Online education platforms** offering CME courses

When approaching potential sponsors, it's helpful to have a media kit that outlines your podcast's audience demographics, listenership numbers, and advertising rates. Be prepared to negotiate the terms of the sponsorship agreement, including the length of the sponsorship, the number of ads per episode, and the level of creative control the sponsor will have. Also, ensure that your listeners are aware of the sponsorship and that you are transparent about any potential conflicts of interest.

Grants and Institutional Funding

If your podcast has an educational focus, consider applying for grants from:

- **Medical foundations and nonprofit organizations** supporting education
- **University and hospital education departments** willing to fund professional development initiatives
- **Governmental and private grants** related to medical communication

Grant writing can be a time-consuming process, but it can be a valuable source of funding for your podcast. Research potential grant opportunities thoroughly and carefully follow the application guidelines. Be sure to highlight the educational value of your podcast and how it aligns with the grant funder's mission.

Listener Support and Crowdfunding

A variety of online platforms allow dedicated listeners to contribute financially. These platforms make it easy for listeners to support your podcast with recurring or one-time donations. Offering exclusive content—such as bonus episodes, live Q&As, or resource guides—can encourage paid subscriptions. Providing valuable perks can incentivize listeners to become paying subscribers.

When setting up a listener support platform, it's important to clearly communicate the value of supporting your podcast. Explain how listener contributions will help you continue to produce high-quality content and improve the listening experience. Also, be sure to thank your supporters publicly and acknowledge their contributions.

Merchandising

In imagining your podcast, you might dream of fans wearing tee shirts and sipping from mugs emblazoned with your logo. Merchandising can be a fun way to engage with your audience and generate additional revenue for your podcast. Depending on how you price branded items, they may simply serve as advertising or even contribute to your cashflow.

Merchandising, however, adds a level of complexity to your endeavor as well. Now you're not only producing and distributing one product—your podcast—you're also in the retail business. That means selecting and sourcing appropriate products, fielding orders for those products, and ensuring they reach your fans. Managing inventory, processing orders, and handling customer service can be time-consuming and challenging. On the accounting side, you may also need to track numbers like inventory and sales tax for accurate reporting.

A wealth of outlets now promises to help with order fulfillment end-to-end, with just-in-time manufacturing to keep inventory from stacking up. Using print-on-demand services eliminates inventory concerns and allows easy fulfillment. These services handle the printing, packaging, and shipping of your merchandise, freeing you from the logistical challenges of running a retail business. At a minimum these services keep you from having to stack boxes of tee shirts in your garage and stuff them in envelopes to ship to your buyers. On the other hand, these firms usually charge based on volume, so if you think your sales will be in the dozens rather than the thousands, they may not prove cost-effective. You will want to vet these vendors carefully, since the products that are going out represent your brand, and when glitches occur the buck will stop with you, figuratively and literally.

Types of Merchandise to Consider:

- **Branded Apparel:** Scrubs, lab coats, T-shirts, and hoodies with your podcast's logo

- **Medical-Themed Accessories:** Notebooks, coffee mugs, or even stethoscope tags featuring your branding
- **Educational Materials:** PDF guides, quick-reference sheets, or digital workbooks based on podcast content
- **Limited-Edition Items:** Special items related to milestones (e.g., "100th Episode" merchandise)

When selecting merchandise, consider your target audience and their interests. Choose products that are relevant to the medical field and that your listeners would be proud to wear or use. Also, be sure to offer a range of sizes and styles to accommodate a diverse audience.

Social Media Promotion

Podcasting is a profoundly online endeavor, so you'll want to build your following online as well. Social media can be a powerful tool for promoting your podcast and engaging with your audience. Not only are you promoting your brand and helping people find you, but you're also building a corps of devoted fans who can help promote your podcast to listeners you'd never reach on your own. Building a strong online community can amplify your podcast's reach and impact. This means engaging your followers actively and regularly.

At first, you may be tempted to spread your brand across every social media platform you can imagine, from Facebook to X to LinkedIn to Bluesky. However, it's often more effective to focus your efforts on a few key platforms where your target audience is most active. Cross-posting can also be limited by the differences in each platform's requirements and format, and you can easily find yourself with yet another full-time job on top of practicing medicine and producing a podcast. Choose the platforms that align best with your content and audience.

In some cases, cross-posting is easy. Meta can coordinate posts across Facebook, Instagram, and Threads, for example. In other cases, you may want to tailor a post for different platforms. Creating platform-specific content can increase engagement and reach. YouTube offers a perfect medium for long-form video and audio, including your entire podcast episode if you choose. You can also create shorter video clips with highlights from the episode. TikTok, on the other hand, might offer you ten minutes of video time, but the platform's viewers may lack the patience to stick around for the whole thing. Instead, create short, engaging videos that capture the essence of your podcast. LinkedIn offers chances to network with others in your field and beyond to garner interest in your voice and expertise. Share articles, insights, and updates related to your podcast's topic.

Regardless of where you post, schedule your posts regularly and check in with your followers. Consistency is key to building a strong social media presence. The more you engage, the higher you rise in the algorithm! Respond to comments, answer questions, and participate in relevant discussions. You might ask followers what topic they'd like to hear about on your podcast or what guests might intrigue them. Soliciting feedback from your audience can help you create content that resonates with them. You can stream live Q&A's with followers to further build your community. Live streams can provide a more personal and interactive way to connect with your audience.

You can also tease upcoming episodes and showcase the best lines from episodes that have already aired. Creating anticipation for upcoming content can drive listenership. Artificial intelligence tools exist that can help you select and promote your best moments. These tools use AI to identify the most engaging moments in your podcast, making it easier to create compelling social media content. Depending on how much time and expertise you have, this may be another place where outsourcing your marketing offers a positive return on investment. Hiring a social media manager can free up your time to focus on creating content.

Search engine optimization (SEO) will be a key component of your social media strategy. Using relevant keywords and hashtags can improve the visibility of your posts. Search hashtags and titles that other people are using around your topic and incorporate them in your post. Consider responding to other people's posts in ways that make it clear you have both expertise and a specific perspective. Sharing your insights and expertise can establish you as a thought leader in your field. Whatever you do, however, don't feed the "trolls!" Engaging with negative comments can be draining and unproductive. An online flame war with someone who will never agree with you will sap your energy and distract from your mission of educating the public and your peers. Focus your energy on creating positive and informative content.

Consider these platforms:

- **X:** For professional discussions and medical education hashtags, but may also draw an abundance of negative comments from "trolls"
- **LinkedIn:** Ideal for networking and engaging with academic institutions
- **Instagram & TikTok:** Best for bite-sized, visually appealing content
- **Facebook Groups:** Great for community-based engagement

Tips for sharing:

- **Share episode highlights:** via short clips, infographics, and key quotes
- **Use Hashtags:** #MedEd, #MedicalPodcast, #FOAMed for better reach
- **Encourage Interaction:** Polls, Q&A sessions, and live discussions
- **Cross-Promotion:** Engage with other podcasters, tag guests, and collaborate with influencers

Consider creating a social media calendar to plan your posts in advance. This can help you stay organized and ensure that you are consistently sharing content. Also, track your social media analytics to see what types of posts are performing best and adjust your strategy accordingly.

Multi-platform Promotion: Expanding Your Reach

While social media is crucial, diversifying your promotional efforts across multiple platforms can significantly expand your podcast's reach. Consider these additional strategies:

- **Website:** Create a dedicated website for your podcast with episode descriptions, show notes, guest bios, and links to subscribe on various platforms
- **Email Marketing:** Build an email list to notify subscribers of new episodes, share exclusive content, and promote upcoming events
- **Guest Appearances:** Appear as a guest on other podcasts in your niche to reach new audiences and promote your own show
- **Medical Conferences:** Present your podcast at medical conferences and workshops to connect with potential listeners in person
- **Collaborations:** Partner with other organizations and influencers in the medical field to cross-promote your podcast

Conclusion

Successfully marketing a medical education podcast requires a holistic approach that integrates professional branding, financial strategies, merchandising, social media engagement, and multi-platform promotion. A well-executed marketing strategy can help you attract a dedicated audience, establish yourself as a thought leader, and achieve your podcasting goals. By implementing these strategies, you can grow your audience, enhance credibility, and ensure long-term success in the ever-evolving digital landscape of medical education. Remember to stay adaptable, experiment with different approaches, and continuously analyze your results to optimize your marketing efforts. The world of podcasting is constantly evolving, so it's essential to stay up to date on the latest trends and best practices.

Chapter 10
The Role of AI in Podcasting for Medical Education

Tony Tarchichi and Microsoft Copilot AI

Introduction

AI is now **augmenting podcast production**, making content creation more efficient and accessible. Artificial Intelligence (AI) is a field of computer science dedicated to developing systems capable of performing tasks that typically require human cognition—such as understanding language, recognizing patterns, learning from experience, and making decisions. The development of the Large Language Models (LLMs) within AI spurs this innovation. LLMs allow AI to produce more coherent, contextually relevant responses, making them particularly valuable in communication-driven settings like education and media. Table 10.1 outlines the

Author's Note: This chapter on AI was written with Microsoft Copilot as the co-author. We thought it would be helpful to discuss how this process went. AI had challenges writing this chapter. The original chapter that was written was very short and AI had to be prompted to add more. With each new iteration, it would leave something else out that I didn't ask to be removed. The references were over 50% wrong with wrong authors noted, as the largest issue. Often the topic and description were correct, and the journal or publication would be correct, but the authors were incorrect. It took time to figure out how to use AI to write a chapter. The chapter also had to be edited with significant attention paid to the amount AI praised itself. AI was effusive in its self-praise and over emphasized the time saved using it. While the time initially saved is valuable, currently AI needs a lot of proofreading of its references and its use of effusive language for itself, which significantly diminishes the time saved.

Disclaimer: Any mention of a specific company is not an endorsement of the company. The human author does not have any associations with any of the companies listed.

Microsoft Copilot AI

T. Tarchichi (✉)
Pediatric Hospital Medicine, Children's Hospital of Pittsburgh, Pittsburgh, PA, USA
e-mail: tarchichitr@upmc.edu

J. Parga-Belinkie et al. (eds.), *Podcasting for Medical Professionals*,
https://doi.org/10.1007/978-3-032-16480-3_10

Table 10.1 AI applications in podcasting for medical education

AI application	Function	Benefit in medical education
AI-assisted script writing	Generates structured content	Saves time
AI-generated post-production notes	Summarizes key points	May enhance learning retention
AI translation	Converts podcasts into multiple languages	Potential for global reach
AI-created podcasts	Fully automated content generation	Provides scalable education

various functions AI can assist with when creating a podcast. These include script writing, post-production work including editing, and translating the podcast to different languages. It is also possible for AI to create podcasts independently without a production team or host. This chapter will outline the functionality of AI for podcast creation and discuss the role of AI generated podcasts in medical education.

AI-Assisted Script Writing

AI-assisted script writing refers to the use of AI tools to ideally help generate structured and informative podcast scripts. These tools can analyze medical literature, clinical guidelines, and user prompts to create content that aligns with educational goals. AI should not replace human input but instead serve as a collaborative partner—streamlining the writing process. Any work performed by AI should be reviewed by the podcast production team or host to ensure accuracy and it is in their voice, tone, and teaching style [1]. Additionally, AI has been known to create false citations of medical literature and is prone to something called hallucinations. Hallucinations are when large language models (LLMs) produce incorrect content in a confident way—again making it essential to have a team of content experts review the scripts. That said, a study published in the *ACM Digital Library* explored how AI enhances podcasting by **automating script writing, reducing production time**, and **ensuring consistency** in educational content [2]. AI-generated scripts were found to be particularly useful in maintaining **structured discussions** and integrating **evidence-based medicine** into podcast episodes.

AI-driven tools like **ChatGPT, Jasper, and Descript** assist in generating podcast scripts by analyzing **medical literature, guidelines, and expert discussions**.

How Humans Can Guide AI to Write Personalized Scripts

To ensure the AI-generated script aligns with your educational goals and personal style, consider the following strategies:

- **Define Clear Learning Objectives**
  Start by identifying what you want your audience to learn. For example:
  - "By the end of this episode, listeners should be able to describe the latest ADA guidelines for Type 2 diabetes."
  - "Explain the pathophysiology of atrial fibrillation in simple terms for early medical students."
    These objectives help the AI focus on relevant content and structure.
- **Provide Context and Tone**
  AI performs best when given detailed prompts. Include:
  - Target audience (e.g., "third-year medical students" or "emergency medicine residents")
  - Tone (e.g., conversational, academic, humorous)
  - Format (e.g., monologue, Q&A, case-based discussion)
    Example Prompt:
    "Write a podcast script for internal medicine residents on managing diabetic ketoacidosis. Use a conversational tone and include a case vignette at the beginning."
- **Use Anchoring Examples**
  If you have a past script or transcript that reflects your style, you can feed it into the AI as a reference. This helps the AI mimic your phrasing, pacing, and structure.
- **Iterate and Refine**
  AI-generated drafts are starting points. Use them to:
  - Add personal anecdotes or clinical pearls
  - Insert clarifying questions or transitions
  - Adjust for flow and emphasis
    You can also ask the AI to revise based on feedback:
    "Make this script more concise and add a summary at the end."
- **Incorporate Evidence-Based Content**
  Use AI to summarize recent guidelines or studies, then integrate those summaries into your script. This ensures your content is both current and accurate.
  Example:
  "Summarize the 2024 ESC guidelines on heart failure in 3 bullet points suitable for a podcast script."
- **Maintain Your Voice**
  Even with AI assistance, your unique voice is what builds trust and engagement. Use AI to handle structure and research, but infuse the script with your personality, humor, and clinical experience.

AI-Generated Post-Podcast Production Notes

AI tools like **Otter.ai and Whisper** transcribe and summarize podcast episodes, creating **structured notes** for learners.

AI tools can generate transcripts, summaries, chapters, and show notes for a podcast episode within minutes. This is a significant time-saver compared to manual notetaking or transcription, which can take hours depending on the length and complexity of the episode. AI transcription tools have improved significantly in handling accents and speech nuances, but they are not infallible. Most platforms recommend human review to correct errors and ensure contextual accuracy. A 2025 study found that AI-generated podcast summaries were generally understandable and engaging, but some included inaccuracies and mispronunciations, which affected trustworthiness [3]. Table 10.2 explains some benefits of AI generated notes of podcasts in medical education.

How to Generate AI-Based Post-Podcast Notes

1. **Transcribe the Podcast**—Use AI transcription tools like Otter.ai.
2. **Summarize Key Points**—AI extracts key takeaways and organizes them into sections. Review and modify them as needed.
3. **Enhance with AI-Generated Timestamps**—Learners can jump to specific sections of the podcast.

AI-Powered Translation and AI Voice Cloning

(a) **Definition of AI-Powered Translation**

(i) AI-powered translation refers to the use of artificial intelligence algorithms to automatically translate text or speech from one language to another. These systems leverage machine learning models, often trained on vast multilingual datasets, to understand context, grammar, and nuances, providing translations that are more accurate and natural-sounding compared to traditional rule-based systems.

Table 10.2 Benefits of AI-generated notes in medical education

Benefit	Description
Accessibility	Supports learners with hearing impairments; provides a written summary to reinforce learning
Efficiency	Saves time for educators and learners
Enhanced retention	Structured summaries reinforce learning

(b) **Definition of AI Voice Cloning**

(i) AI voice cloning is the process of using artificial intelligence to create a synthetic replica of a person's voice. This technology can generate speech that mimics the tone, pitch, accent, and speaking style of the original speaker. Voice cloning typically involves training deep learning models on audio recordings of the target voice, enabling the AI to produce new speech outputs that sound remarkably like the original.

AI Translations

AI-driven translation tools like **DeepL and Google Translate** enable podcasts to reach a **global audience**. AI voice cloning maintains **speaker identity across translations**, improving engagement and accessibility. There is a caveat that there are certain languages where AI is significantly less fluent then professional translators, such as Haitian Creole [4].

AI Voice Cloning Tools

Tool	Features
Descript (overdub)	Creates a digital clone of a speaker's voice
ElevenLabs	Ultra-realistic AI-generated voices with multilingual support
Podcastle	High-quality AI-generated speech for professional podcasting
Speechify	Supports over 40 languages with free AI voice cloning

Several studies have examined the impact of AI-powered voice cloning in medical education. A study published in *SpringerLink* explored the evolution of AI voice cloning technologies and their applications in healthcare [5]. Researchers compared traditional rule-based speech synthesis models with modern deep learning systems such as WaveNet, Tacotron, and Transformer-TTS. These newer models significantly improved speech quality, making AI-generated voices almost indistinguishable from human speech. Extrapolating from this study, AI voice cloning could enhance medical education podcasts, improve patient communication, and serve as an assistive technology. However, the researchers also emphasized ethical concerns regarding voice replication and the potential for misuse, advocating for regulatory oversight in AI-generated speech applications.

Further behavioral research conducted by *Cambridge Open Engage* examined human perception of AI-generated voices [6]. Participants listened to synthetic voices and rated them on naturalness and similarity to human speech using

MUSHRA and similarity tests. The findings revealed that AI models like ElevenLabs closely mimicked human-like speech, achieving high ratings for clarity and authenticity. However, models like XTTS and StyleTTS scored lower due to limitations in prosody and rhythm, suggesting that emotional expression and conversational flow still require refinement. The study concluded that AI voice cloning is highly effective for educational applications, but continued improvements in speech dynamics are necessary to fully match human expressiveness.

Collectively, these studies highlight the potential of AI voice cloning in medical education. However, challenges such as ethical considerations, emotional authenticity, and regulatory oversight must be addressed to ensure responsible implementation. Due to the rapidity with which AI is being developed and implemented, these ethical concerns must be addressed as quickly as possible. The most appropriate group to address these concerns through regulation is governments [7, 8]. While you, someone who uses AI, will likely not be in a position to personally regulate AI, we are highlighting these issues as they are the pressing issues we face with AI in the near future. We present some of them below.

Ethical Implications of AI Voice Cloning

While AI voice cloning offers significant benefits, it also raises important ethical considerations:

- **Consent:**
  - It is crucial to obtain explicit consent from individuals before cloning their voice. This ensures respect for personal autonomy and prevents unauthorized use.
- **Identity Misuse:**
  - Voice cloning technology can be misused to impersonate individuals, leading to potential identity theft or fraud. Safeguards must be in place to prevent such misuse.
- **Deepfakes:**
  - The creation of deepfake audio, where AI-generated voices are used to create misleading or harmful content, is a growing concern. This can undermine trust in audio content and have serious repercussions in medical education and beyond.
- **Regulatory Oversight:**
  - There is a need for clear regulations and guidelines governing the use of AI voice cloning. This includes establishing standards for consent, usage, and accountability to ensure ethical practices.
- **Transparency:**
  - It is important to disclose when AI voice cloning is used in podcasting. Transparency helps maintain trust with the audience and ensures they are aware of the technology being used.

By addressing these ethical implications, we can harness the benefits of AI voice cloning while mitigating potential risks.

AI-Created Podcasts: Comprehensive Step-by-Step Guide

AI-created podcasts are audio episodes generated with minimal human input using artificial intelligence tools. These tools can automate nearly every step of the podcast production process—including script writing, voice narration, editing, and even background music—by leveraging natural language processing, text-to-speech synthesis, and audio enhancement technologies. Unlike traditional podcasts, which require human hosts, recording equipment, and manual editing, AI-created podcasts can be produced quickly and at scale, making them ideal for educational content that needs frequent updates or multilingual distribution.

How Can I Make AI-Created Podcasts?

Step 1: Define the Podcast Topic and Format

- Choose a **medical education topic** (e.g., "Cardiology Case Studies")
- Decide on the format (e.g., monologue, interview-style, case discussion)

Step 2: Generate the Script Using AI

- Use **ChatGPT, Jasper, or Descript** to create a structured script.

Step 3: Convert Text to Speech Using AI Voice Generation

Tool	Features
Podcastle	Over 1000 AI voices with customizable accents
VEED.IO	Converts text into podcasts with AI-generated narration
Descript (overdub)	Allows digital voice cloning for corrections
ElevenLabs	Ultra-realistic multilingual AI-generated voices

Step 4: Add AI-Generated Background Music and Sound Effects

Tool	Features
Sonify	AI-generated soundscapes
Giz.AI	Creates high-quality audio samples
DeepAI music generator	Produces customized AI-generated music

Step 5: Edit and Enhance Using AI Audio Processing

- **Use Adobe Podcast or VEED.IO** for **background noise removal, clarity enhancement**, and **final touch-ups**.

Step 6: Publish and Distribute

- Upload to **Spotify, Apple Podcasts**, or **YouTube**.
- Use AI-powered analytics tools to track listener engagement.

Recent research and industry analyses have explored the impact of AI-generated podcasts compared to traditional podcasts, highlighting differences in efficiency, authenticity, and audience engagement. A report from *Jellypod* emphasizes that AI-generated podcasts streamline production by automating scripting, editing, and distribution while maintaining high content quality [9]. However, the report underscores that traditional podcasts still hold an advantage in human connection, storytelling, and spontaneity, elements that AI-generated content currently struggles to replicate.

For medical education podcasts that are made for-profit an understanding of the financial considerations for AI generated podcasts is essential. A separate industry analysis published by *Bm Times* examines why many entrepreneurs and businesses are shifting toward AI-driven podcasting. AI tools enhance audio processing, transcription, content repurposing, and SEO optimization, making podcast production more efficient and scalable. Businesses that rely on frequent podcast publishing benefit from AI's ability to automate content creation while maintaining professional sound quality. However, traditional podcasts continue to be favored in fields that require deep discussions, interviews, and dynamic interaction between hosts and guests, areas where AI-generated voices may lack natural variability and emotional depth.

Additionally, *Podcast Hawk* has investigated whether AI-generated podcasts are disrupting traditional broadcasting. The analysis suggests that AI-driven content is reshaping media consumption by producing personalized news, educational materials, and entertainment. AI-powered automation assists with editing, mixing, and real-time translation, making podcasts more accessible across multiple languages. However, the report raises concerns about creativity and originality, noting that AI-generated scripts sometimes lack the nuanced perspectives and improvisational depth that human hosts bring to discussions.

Overall, while AI-generated podcasts offer advantages in efficiency, scalability, and automation, traditional podcasts remain superior in fostering audience engagement, emotional connection, and conversational flow. The future of podcasting in medical education will likely involve a hybrid approach—leveraging AI to enhance production and accessibility while preserving human-led discussions for deeper learning experiences.

Conclusion

AI is transforming podcasting in medical education by **streamlining content creation, enhancing accessibility, and expanding global reach**. While AI-generated podcasts offer **efficiency and scalability**, human-led podcasts remain essential for **engagement and nuanced discussions**. The future will likely see a hybrid approach, leveraging AI for **efficiency while maintaining human expertise** for depth and connection.

References

1. Colasacco CJ, Born HL. A case of artificial intelligence Chatbot hallucination. JAMA Otolaryngol Neck Surg. 2024;150(6):457–8. https://doi.org/10.1001/jamaoto.2024.0428.
2. Samuel AAA. Enhancing podcasting by Leveraging AI Technologies. Accessed June 26, 2025. https://dl.acm.org/doi/fullHtml/10.1145/3626767.3625304
3. Desmedt CP, Budts W, De Vos M, Moons P. Artificial intelligence-generated podcasts open new doors to make science accessible: a mixed-method evaluation of quality and the potential for science communication. Eur J Cardiovasc Nurs. Published online June 14, 2025:zvaf074. https://doi.org/10.1093/eurjcn/zvaf074.
4. Brewster RCL, Gonzalez P, Khazanchi R, et al. Performance of ChatGPT and Google translate for pediatric discharge instruction translation. Pediatrics. 2024;154(1):e2023065573. https://doi.org/10.1542/peds.2023-065573.
5. Patel AK, Madnani H, Tripathi S, Sharma P, Shukla VK. Real-time voice cloning: artificial intelligence to clone and generate human voice. In: Hasteer N, Blum C, Mehrotra D, Pandey HM, editors. Intelligent solutions for smart adaptation in digital era. Springer Nature; 2025. p. 349–64. https://doi.org/10.1007/978-981-97-8193-5_29.
6. Bakkouche L, Cooper S, Luo X, et al. Finding the human voice in AI: insights on the perception of AI-voice clones from MUSHRA and similarity tests. Published online November 14, 2024. https://doi.org/10.33774/coe-2024-mvrz5.
7. Alafgani J. Automated Podcast Creation: Produce Professional Podcasts Without the Hassle. October 29, 2024. Accessed June 26, 2025. https://jellypod.ai/blog/automated-podcast-creation
8. Aziz T. AI vs. Traditional Podcasting: Why Smart Entrepreneurs Are Making the Switch? Bm Times. March 26, 2025. Accessed June 26, 2025. https://bmtimes.co.uk/ai-vs-traditional-podcasting-why-smart-entrepreneursare-making-the-switch/
9. Townsend S. Are AI generated Podcasts Disrupting Traditional Broadcasting? Podcast Hawk. December 2, 2024. Accessed June 26, 2025. https://podcasthawk.com/are-ai-generated-podcasts-disrupting-traditionalbroadcasting/

Chapter 11
Podcasting in an Academic Career

Katie Lockwood

Introduction

The entertaining nature of podcasts often leads to an underappreciation of this medium as a form of academic scholarship. Yet, medical podcasts require a scholarly investment from all participants. The podcast producer, host, and guest all contribute academically to podcast creation. The producer needs an understanding of the topic to find an expert guest. The host must have extensive background knowledge on the subject to generate thoughtful and well-designed interview questions. Lastly, the guest requires the balance of knowing the information to answer the questions and the ability to deliver it in an entertaining and efficient manner. A successful podcast episode sounds like a casual conversation between experts on a topic of interest to all, but is more often a well-orchestrated, over-researched, and semi-scripted academic dialogue. Put simply, it is work. Work that is like all other scholarly work that academic healthcare providers engage in. It therefore should be given equal value on *curriculum vitae,* faculty promotion applications, and considerations for funding by institutions.

Podcasts on *Curriculum Vitae*

Where a podcast fits on a *curriculum vitae* (CV) may vary depending on the individual formatting, but what is clear is that they belong. Podcasts are a form of multimedia included in the American Medical Association (AMA) Manual of Style, 11th edition [1], which states that podcasts can be cited as:

K. Lockwood (✉)
Department of Pediatrics, Children's Hospital of Philadelphia, Philadelphia, PA, USA
e-mail: lockwoodk@chop.edu

J. Parga-Belinkie et al. (eds.), *Podcasting for Medical Professionals*,
https://doi.org/10.1007/978-3-032-16480-3_11

Last Name First Initial. Podcast Title. Episode Title. Date Published. Date Accessed. URL.

Many choose to list podcasts under "Publications" on their CV, but this section may also be subdivided into sections including peer reviewed papers, review articles, book chapters, editorials, podcasts, etc. Many podcast guests will be first timers and may not know podcasts can be cited as scholarly work, so it is important for podcast producers and/or hosts to remind them and provide the citation for their episode. In doing so, more podcast episodes will appear on CVs, shifting the culture towards using podcasts for academic promotion.

If a healthcare provider serves as a podcast producer, host, editor, or other essential role, it is important to list this role on the CV as well. In medicine these additional roles in podcasting are often taken on as "side gigs" and passion projects, forgetting that these are professional roles. The skills required to be a producer, host, or editor are skills that have been earned and are translatable to other careers. This role should be listed on a CV along with other academic positions held, and in featuring it as so, demonstrates its rigor and time investment.

Podcasts and Academic Promotion

Traditionally, scholarship for academic promotion has included peer-reviewed publications, invited talks, grants, Continuing Medical Education (CME) curricula, academic committee participation, and editorial roles. Digital and social media were not historically viewed in a scholarly context. Mayo Clinic emerged as a leader in 2016 when they considered digital and social media scholarship among the criteria considered for academic advancement by their Academic Appointments and Promotions Committee [2].

Some of the pre-production scholarly work of podcasting can be harder to quantify in terms of impact, but just as a journal editorial role would be captured in an academic promotion application, so should the editor-in-chief of a clinical podcast. Cabrera et al. [2] suggest an impact grid for institutions to assess podcast scholarship for an editor-in-chief role on a clinical podcast with 2000 downloads/views per month as low impact, 5000 downloads/views per month as medium impact, and 20,000 downloads/view per month as high impact. Using a standardized approach such as an impact grid for podcast scholarship can help academic promotions committee members who are less familiar with this medium assess the impact factor and give appropriate credit to these roles.

Another aspect of impact is global reach. Traditionally, academic promotion included giving invited talks that escalated from local/regional to national to international, representing an escalating esteem and reach of one's academic reputation. With podcasts, talented teachers and medical communicators can easily reach audiences beyond their home institution. Podcasters are also able to collect detailed demographic data on the listener audience, including country [3]. Through podcasting, an academic may be able to reach an international audience through a widely disseminated podcast episode, oftentimes with a much larger audience than any in person invited lecture would have in attendance [4].

Podcasters should describe their work in their portfolio using Glassick's framework [2, 5]:

- Clear goals
- Adequate preparation
- Appropriate methods
- Significant results
- Effective presentation
- Reflective technique

Within this framework, podcasters can explore how: podcasts are used for medical education, the amount of research and preparation involved in pre-production, the structured interview methods used, captured data metrics, feedback data on presentation, and reflection on the meritorious nature of podcasting in medical education. Using a structure allows committee members to compare podcasters to other medical educators in a standardized manner.

Additional places podcasts may appear in academic promotion applications include in mentoring of trainees in podcast production, research related to podcasts, or as an invited lectures as a podcast guest contributor. Furthermore, podcasting can be highlighted as an innovative approach to education in academic clinician tracks. Podcasters can highlight the reach of their episodes compared to traditional educational platforms such as Grand Rounds or webinars, the diversity of guest contributors, and the asynchronous nature, which allows for greater learner autonomy in choosing the right time and place for education. Informal or non-traditional data can also be collected, such as ratings and reviews from iTunes or Spotify, feedback from guest contributors, or data on referrals that resulted from podcast listens. Podcasting represents an important educational niche that adds value to the academic clinician track by diversifying how we deliver education, expanding education beyond the walls of our institutions, and exposing our audience to a wider variety of educators than possible at the local level.

Podcast episodes can vary greatly in style, content, and quality. As difficult as it is for listeners to discern a high-yield medical podcast, it may be even more challenging for promotions committees to evaluate the scholarship of podcasts with traditional academic output. Therefore, Helton and Pathman[6] used a mini-Delphi approach to reach consensus on seven criteria to evaluate whether a faculty work product counts as scholarship toward promotion.

These Helton and Pathman [6] criteria included:

- Expertise: faculty member's expertise
- Faculty contribution: degree of meaningful engagement
- Originality: new information, insights, or methods
- Peer review: impartially evaluated
- Quality: carefully prepared, organized, written

- Relative permanence: accessible to others for at least 3 years
- Impact: accessed by others beyond one's home campus and influenced the field

Although some subjectivity in application is expected and not all criteria need to be met, these criteria give a framework to assess podcasts in terms of scholarly impact for promotion. In a field where it seems anyone can have a podcast, this framework helps identify those that count towards scholarship, which can be helpful for both podcast creators and guests who submit content for faculty promotion.

Another element often identified in promotion packages is mentorship of trainees and podcasting offers ample opportunity to promote trainee scholarship. Trainees are eager to become involved in podcasting as this is a medium with which they often engage for their own education. Trainees can join on an episodic basis, getting involved with a particular topic, or longitudinally in creating multiple episodes. Many podcasts have a history of heavy trainee involvement, including *PedsCases, Short White Coat*, and *Cribsiders*, where attendings mentor trainees through the process of episode production but trainees are involved in and accountable for all aspects of development, production, and post-production. Other podcasts like *Primary Care Perspectives by the Children's Hospital of Philadelphia* may have trainees as episode guests when they are content experts, but they are not regularly involved in production. The mentorship of trainees in podcasting though can lead to scholarly output of podcast episodes as well as potential for research, embedding podcasts in residency curriculum, and ongoing mentoring relationships.

Academics can also consider the formal adoption of podcasting knowledge and skills into the medical curriculum for trainees. An example of this can be found at the Children's Hospital of Philadelphia. There senior residents can elect to take an Advanced Skills course, which is a longitudinal elective they complete over two years of their pediatric training. Such an advanced skills course was developed in podcasting to allow for a deeper understanding of the scholarship surrounding this medium. Over two years, residents engage in lectures, direct observation, and mentoring to build skills to meet their desired podcasting learning objectives. The goal is to generate at least one podcast episode, but learners can go further. They can become producers, guests, hosts, or occupy a combination of roles, and feel confident in applying those skills again in the future to incorporate into their career. At graduation, these residents receive a certificate in Advanced Skills in Podcasting, a novel award that makes these residents part of a small, but growing, cohort of pediatric podcasters. Incorporating podcasting skill-building into graduate medical education offers trainees the opportunity to compete in the modern digital technology education workforce. It also allows faculty who develop these curricula to develop an educational niche within the graduate medical education landscape.

More broadly than academic promotion, podcasting faces a challenge of institutional support that includes funding of time enabling academic clinicians to engage in this work. Like any scholarly work, academic clinicians need time away from patient care responsibilities to engage in the pre-production work, as well as have recording time. Many academic clinicians receive funded time more generally for education or research, but podcasting is rarely considered in either of these traditional funding streams or bundled together with other educational demands. Podcasters should try to seek funding for podcasting specifically but may need to think creatively about where that funding is from.

Funding a Podcast

It is difficult for institutions to quantify the impact of a podcast to justify the investment of this funding. However, metrics are available including number of downloads, demographics of listeners, and engagement with episodes. In looking for funding support it is important for the clinician and the institution to consider the goals of the podcast and the intended audience. Funding may come from the division level to meet education needs but may also be more appropriate from public relations or marketing, physician engagement and outreach, government affairs, or similar departments within an institution. For example, an educational podcast about diabetes geared toward residents and fellows may fall under the education budget of graduate medical education or the Division of Endocrinology. Whereas a podcast about advocacy efforts of clinicians and their impact on patients may fall under funding from the marketing or government affairs office. Oftentimes podcasts receive mixed sources of funding, with resources being funded by public relations or marketing and their time being funded through their division. If a podcast is focused on practicing providers, funds earmarked for faculty development or CME may be appropriate to use for podcast funding. Rather, if a podcast is focused on trainee education, funds may be solicited from an affiliated college of medicine or other professional school to help support trainee education.

Institutions may also have institutional grants, foundation funding, or private donors, who are willing to fund podcasts on specific topics. Podcasters may need to meet with representatives from public relations, marketing, and development, to determine the most appropriate and available funding streams. Podcasters may consider community or national grants, university research grants, or CME-funding as alternative funding streams.

As mentioned earlier in this book, some podcast funding can be achieved through advertisers. This approach should be considered with caution for academic podcasts to ensure that there is no bias at play and that advertisers do not pose a conflict with institutional policies.

Institutional and Other Affiliations

In creating a podcast, there are pros and cons of being affiliated with an institution. The greatest benefit may be funding of non-clinical time and coverage of podcast expenses. The institution can sometimes help provide supplementary support for podcasting skills that a healthcare provider may not have, such as marketing or sound editing. A downside though is the loss of creative control and need to adhere to institutional standards. For example, the institution may dictate what content is covered or what guests are featured. Institutional podcasts need to adhere to a professional standard, meaning there should not be cursing, commercial bias, or an overly casual tone. The institution may also own the intellectual property and if the podcast became successful, it will not be a potential revenue stream for the podcast host but rather the institution.

In having an independently sponsored podcast, the individual retains creative control and intellectual property rights (depending on the institutional contract) but will be responsible for finding funding streams and fulfilling all technical roles. Even if independent, it is wise to make the institution aware of the affiliation with the podcast, as healthcare providers represent their institutions whether implicitly or explicitly. The institution and the healthcare provider can then determine if it is best for the provider to disclose their institutional title or not in their podcasting role. However, once independence is established, the podcast host can take the podcast wherever they please. Independent podcasts often are more personal, covering topics like fitness, personal finance, travel, and mental health. These podcasters can choose whichever guests they like, regardless of institutional affiliation or loyalties, and promote products or services that may not be endorsed by their home institution. There is also the possibility for generating revenue from these podcasts, as some of the more prominent podcasters have been able to achieve. Notably though if podcasters are making revenue this could become a conflict of interest and constitute a relevant disclosure as such.

Beyond partnering with a home institution, podcasting partnerships can be formed with another healthcare company, such as a non-profit, community group, medical journal, advocacy organization, or medical industry or device company. In exploring these roles, podcasters should consider how this affiliation might promote bias or conflict of interest in their professional role. Partnering with professional organizations can be an ideal way to look for support outside a home institution but within an organization whose mission aligns with the same professional goals, such as the *Pediatrics On Call* and *Healthy Children* podcasts from American Academy of Pediatrics, *Bedside Rounds* podcast supported by the American College of Physicians, and the *KeyLIME+ podcast* from the Royal College of Physicians and Surgeons of Canada.

Podcasts have an increasingly large presence in medical journals, including the New England Journal of Medicine (NEJM) and the Journal of the American Medical Association (JAMA), and at national conferences. Many institutions now feature their hospital-based podcasts as part of their marketing campaigns. Live podcasting at conferences has become a way to generate excitement for podcasts and allow audiences to meet the hosts, as well as further legitimizing podcasts as a form of academic scholarship.

Institutional Benefits of Podcasting

Institutions understand medical podcasts have an eager audience. Whether its patients looking for health information or healthcare professionals engaging in ongoing education, medical podcasts continue to grow in popularity. Those branded by trusted healthcare institutions gain instant credibility, which is an important quality indicator in podcasts [7]. An institutional podcast can align medical education with institutional goals for recruitment, referrals, and brand recognition. While listening to an educational episode, podcast audiences may learn about career opportunities, specialty programs, or diagnostic centers, of which they were not previously aware. This can generate new sources of engagement with the institution. Having an institutional-branded podcast can also drive consumer traffic to institutional websites and become a source of patient referrals, particularly for tertiary and quaternary care centers who rely on increasing awareness of subspecialty and research programs.

Beyond brand recognition, podcasting can dismantle institutional silos and foster interdisciplinary collaboration. Podcast development may require the cooperation of clinicians, public relations, marketing, web development, legal, and other teams, who may not otherwise have worked together in a team-based manner. In addition, podcast producers, hosts, and guests may cross disciplines and in the process of engaging in podcast content development spread awareness within an institution of programs and services that would not otherwise be known. Podcasts also offer the unique opportunity within medicine for an alternative to the traditional hierarchical structure. For example, an attending physician may not be the most expert or senior in the podcasting domain and medical students may be the leaders as is the case with the *Short White Coat* podcast. For these reasons, institutions should consider the benefits of supporting their own podcasts both internally and externally.

Conclusion

Podcast creation offers faculty development opportunities for the production team, guests, and listeners and is increasingly being included in faculty promotion committee reviews using standardized frameworks. In funding podcasts and podcaster time, institutions support a medium that allows for interprofessional education, collaboration, and brand recognition. While funding streams may be complex, institutional funding not only shows support, but allows academic podcasts to exist without commercial bias or advertisers thus gaining the credibility and trust of audiences. While some podcasters may be eager to work with institutions for their support, many have found challenges and barriers in academic medicine that have led them to operate outside of academia. In the modern digital landscape with the overwhelming appeal of online influencers, digital education, and clickbait culture, institutions should want to claim podcasters as brand ambassadors. These podcasters are leaders in education innovation, skilled spokespeople, and often, healthcare celebrities. Podcasters bring academic merit and entertainment to the stale world of patient education and CME and advocacy is needed for these unique medical education skills to be highly valued by academic institutions.

References

1. Iverson C, editor. American Medical Association manual of style: a guide for authors and editors. 11th ed. Oxford University Press; 2020.
2. Cabrera D, Vartabedian BS, Spinner RJ, Jordan BL, Aase LA, Timimi FK. More than likes and tweets: creating social media portfolios for academic promotion and tenure. J Grad Med Educ. 2017;9:421–5.
3. Rodman A, Trivedi S. Podcasting: a roadmap to the future of medical education. Semin Nephrol. 2020;40:279–83.
4. Parga-Belinkie JJ, Cosmini M, Hill D, Berk J, Lockwood K, Patrick M, Novak C, Tarchichi TR. The role of medical education podcasts in pediatrics. Pediatrics. 2023;152(5):e2023062911. https://doi.org/10.1542/peds.2023-062911.
5. Glassick CE. Boyer's expanded definitions of scholarship, the standards for assessing scholarship, and the elusiveness of the scholarship of teaching. Acad Med. 2000 Sep;75(9):877–80.
6. Helton MR, Pathman DE. Scholarship criteria for promotion in the age of diverse faculty roles and digital media. Fam Med. 2023;55(8):544–6.
7. Lin M, Thoma B, Trueger NS, Ankel F, Sherbino J, Chan T. Quality indicators for blogs and podcasts used in medical education: modified Delphi consensus recommendations by an international cohort of health professions educators. Postgrad Med J. 2015;91(1080):546–50.

Chapter 12
Integration of Podcasts in Curricula

Sara W. Dong

Introduction

As medical education podcasts have grown in popularity, educators are faced with the challenge of how to best appraise and incorporate podcasts into their teaching. Although research on the best approach of using podcasts for learning is still limited, available literature supports that podcasts are well-received by learners and can leverage various educational strategies that align with adult learning theory. A scoping review of podcast use in medical education found that podcasts are highly valued among learners, demonstrate noninferiority compared with traditional teaching methods, and are associated with self-reported practice changes among residents and practicing physicians [1]. Adapting podcasts into educational initiatives or curricula requires planning of both appropriate content curation and strategies for integration. Strategies that transform audio podcast files from passive learning to interactive experiences offer opportunities to increase knowledge retention as well as engagement in synchronous teaching sessions.

Curating Podcast Episodes

The foundation for effective integration of podcasts into teaching is thoughtful curation of materials that align with learning objectives.

S. W. Dong (✉)
Division of Infectious Diseases, Beth Israel Deaconess Medical Center, Boston Children's Hospital, Harvard Medical School, Boston, MA, USA

J. Parga-Belinkie et al. (eds.), *Podcasting for Medical Professionals*,
https://doi.org/10.1007/978-3-032-16480-3_12

Determine Goals and Align with Learning Objectives

Before initiating any planned educational experience, it is important to outline the intended goals and objectives of a session or larger curriculum. A framework such as Kern's six step approach for curriculum development provides a practical guide that can assist in this process, particularly steps one through four [2]. In Step 1, a problem identification and general needs assessment will give insight into the potential needs of a learner community. What knowledge, skills, attitudes should a student gain? What knowledge gap or problem can this project or curriculum address? Reflection on these needs can then shape the overarching goal of the curriculum.

Educators can begin to craft a curriculum development strategy that aligns content and the desired integration of resources by conducting a subsequent targeted needs assessment (Step 2) of learners and stakeholders. Who is the target audience, and which methods or resources may work best? Once the needs of this group have been clarified, educators will have a sound basis to create both broad general goals and specific measurable objectives (Step 3). Pre-existing materials can be curated based on whether they fill an existing gap or serve a complementary purpose to other educational materials in the curriculum. Step 4 focuses on selection of content and understanding what methods would be most likely to achieve the educational objectives. This step is critical as it requires not just identifying podcasts as a modality but considering which educational strategy will be used with the episode or excerpt. The principles of this framework can be used to prepare simpler one-time activities, guide creation of podcast repositories, or drive more comprehensive curricula. Materials will then benefit from iterative review to ensure ongoing alignment with learning objectives.

Familiarize Oneself with Available Podcasts

Once the goals and learning objectives have been clarified, educators can seek out possible podcast resources. The volume of podcast material may seem overwhelming, but various considerations can help narrow down the field and assist in selecting with intention amongst pre-existing resources.

Consider the style and type of medical education podcast that might align best with curricular goals. Formats can vary, such as a monologue with a single host compared to conversation or interview style with multiple speakers. Podcasts may vary in style from casual and conversational to more narrative with heavier emphasis on editing. The length of an episode may be an important consideration, although educators can also select specific excerpts to provide to learners. Listening to a wide variety of podcasts also helps to better understand the various types of information that may be discussed, which can range from models of clinical reasoning and diagnosis to multidisciplinary expert reviews and analysis of recent research. One of the unique strengths of podcasts and other digital education formats is the ability to incorporate less "traditional" topics and varied perspectives from patients or multidisciplinary healthcare professional team members. Seek out podcasts that feature diverse perspectives and discuss topics that are not commonly found or addressed in textbooks or standard didactic teaching sessions, such as ethics, medical humanities, or antiracism.

In addition to personal search, solicit recommendations from other educators as well as the intended learners. Word-of-mouth still remains an important method to hear about relevant and commonly used resources in the educational community. When receiving a recommendation, inquire about why they use and enjoy the podcast. Other forums where you might identify relevant podcasts might include specialty/subspecialty conferences, national organizations or working groups, or social media. Some of the podcasts that might be relevant may even be created by individuals or workgroups representing national or international organizations and journals.

Assess Quality

Definitions of quality for educational podcasts have not been clearly standardized, and unfortunately the gestalt of an individual educator is not a reliable marker of quality [3]. Although there are no validated instruments, various frameworks and tools exist that can provide educators insight and structure for evaluating quality, such as through checklists [4–9]. An overview of general quality considerations are summarized by categories below.

Accessibility, Functionality, and Design Does the podcast utilize a platform that is universally available to allow any learner with standard equipment and software to access? Are technical aspects such as audio delivery clear? Learners benefit from the autonomy of podcasts including the freedom to review a desired topic at a time, place, and pace that is convenient for them. The ability to accelerate playback or pause to process, repeat or research topics of interest is an important component of interfacing with podcast software that can leverage cognitive learning strategies and improve the learners' perception of the experience [10–14]. It also provides increased access for learners who may speak English as a second language.

Content, Academic Rigor, and Professionalism Is the information presented accurate and consistent with current medical evidence and guidelines? Does the podcast provide the appropriate amount of background knowledge to situate the learner and cover an appropriate amount of information for its length? Is it well written, organized, and formatted? Carefully selecting podcast length and complexity helps manage cognitive load and supports knowledge integration [15].

Credibility, Bias, and Transparency Does the podcast provide and cite its references? Are the references mapped to specific statements? Is the identity of the resource author clear, and is that author well qualified to provide information on the topic? Are there clear disclosures of any conflicts of interest? Is there clear differentiation between advertisement versus content and fact versus opinion?

Editorial Processes Is there use of a defined editorial or pre-publication peer review process? Is there evidence of the ability to provide post-publication commentary and discussion?

Other Considerations Evaluate if there are associated resources with the podcast such as a website with show notes (written summaries of the key learning points and references), transcripts, and possible visual communications (such as infographics or visual summaries, educational videos). These resources can provide learners with more ways to interact with content. Alternatively, you may consider what local resources might pair well if there are not pre-existing materials created with the podcast.

Organize Content by Theme or Rotation

Organization of the curated podcast material can follow various structures depending on the program and curriculum needs. Some examples may include collections based on rotation, topic, and progressive complexity. Rotation-based collections are useful when episodes are curated relevant to specific clinical rotations, where trainees can find focused content at the point of clinical exposure. Topic-based collections can organize episodes around core topics or competencies, which can serve as comprehensive learning modules and are also easy to sort based on clinical exposures. If this material is being used across multilevel learner teams, progressive complexity collections may help. Episodes could be structured in complexity from foundational concepts to more advanced nuances, supporting learners across training levels.

Plan for Implementation

Transforming podcast listening from a passive to an active learning experience requires planning. Key strategies and best practices can be based on evidence-based cognitive learning strategies, whether podcasts are incorporated in clinical teaching on-the-fly or into formalized educational structures.

Learner Orientation & Listening Guidance

Before assigning a podcast for learning, an educator should prompt and orient learners to the purpose of the listening experience. Clearly state the purpose of the activity and share specific learning goals. The established goals of the activity can guide learners as they listen and interpret information. Encourage learners to concentrate on the speaker(s) and strive to understand the intended meaning without judgment or bias. Other strategies may include active note-taking strategies, which can pinpoint critical learning points. Educators should provide a clear time commitment for the activity, which may be the length of a full episode or a clearly defined excerpt. The final piece is to explain how you plan to follow-up or assess the listening activity. Consider developing some focused guided questions and when you may provide supplementary resources.

Setting these expectations can supply learners with structure to get the most from their listening experience. Active or "attentive" listening has been described as a cognitive and active process that includes interpretation, and providing this as context can shape the listening process [16, 17]. The additional benefit of deep listening skills is the translation into enhanced clinical experiences with better rapport, minimized misunderstandings, and improved communication of treatment plans [17–19]. While learners may naturally focus on content first, educators can guide listener attention to additional features of an audio recording such as speaker word choice or tone. These non-word features of spoken language (referred to as paralanguage) can provide clues to the emotional states and attitudes of a speaker towards a topic [16]. For example, this may be relevant if the podcast is used to share a narrative piece of a first-person patient experience.

Follow-Up & Expand

Embrace Cognitive Learning Strategies

Educators can use various evidence-based practices to improve learning, which can be built purposefully into a clinical teaching plan or a curriculum. A group of cognitive psychologists who study memory, attention, and perception have previously identified essential strategies, and understanding these mechanisms can illustrate how an educator may build podcasts into a learning activity or curriculum [20–23]. These strategies can be employed together or separately.

1. Spaced practice [24–26] and interleaving [25, 27, 28]: Spaced practice is a strategy of distributing learning sessions over time to improve learning. Calling information to mind again several weeks after first learning improves long-term retention. Interleaving also involves spacing out material, but jumbling or alternating similar concepts in a different order adds an additional benefit, especially for comparing and contrasting topics. Depending on how podcasts are built into

a curriculum, episodes could be spaced out over time or used in combination with other techniques (such as quizzes, writing exercises, or reviewing other materials) to improve learning.

2. Elaboration [29, 30] and concrete examples: Elaboration expands details around a concept by incorporating "why" and "how" questions which build comprehension beyond the knowledge base of just simple facts. This technique is particularly helpful for more advanced learners to create connections and solidify understanding. Abstract concepts can also be solidified with use of varied concrete examples. Podcasts are an excellent tool to provide expanded discussions and alternative scenarios. Learners can then associate a concept with varied aspects and seek similarities and connections. For example, clinical reasoning podcasts can be particularly effective at expanding a learner's library of diagnostic schemas or illness scripts, which can spark a robust discussion on rounds or in a classroom session.
3. Dual coding: Combining visual and verbal information will improve retention, but educators must be selective of what is included to ensure it adds value as redundant information can hamper learning. Consider how supplemental written or visual materials may be used alongside or separate from the assigned audio podcasts.
4. Retrieval practice [31]: Retrieval practice prioritizes active recall over passive recall by bringing a topic back to mind. Quizzes can act as simple knowledge checks to solidify knowledge. Debriefs or discussions about a topic may also provide an opportunity to review content. Digital tools such as online flashcards or scheduled emails/reminders may be another way to assist this method.

Engagement Methods

The simplest method of utilizing podcasts in a live classroom session is to directly play a small audio excerpt to a class. This excerpt can provide a basis for reflection and discussion amongst the group of class members. Other simple models would be creating libraries or collections of podcast episodes that align with modular curriculums or clinical rotations, which learners can easily access and self-select.

A more interactive model for using podcasts would be the flipped classroom. In the flipped classroom model, podcasts (as well as other video, audio, or text resources) are assigned for self-directed pre-class preparation and foundational content delivery, while the in-person synchronous session time focuses on engaging with application, discussion, and problem-solving among peers. This method can be implemented as elements in an individual session or built throughout an entire team-based learning curriculum. Use of a flipped classroom method among health professional learners has been shown to lead to improvement in student learning, creation of environments of inquiry and open questioning, and was preferred over traditional lectures [32–36].

Pre-class or session preparation can be prepared as noted in the Learner Orientation & Listening Guidance section previously. The face-to-face or in-classroom phase may incorporate facilitated discussion and reflection, case-based instruction, simulation, peer instruction, or problem-solving activities that apply and extend concepts introduced in the podcast. The type of active learning exercise should be selected or designed to align with the intended goal or competency. Some examples might include:

- Provide a podcast related to a clinical topic. During the in-class phase, facilitate discussion such as comparison of case features to prior clinical experiences or discussion of challenges in management. Strategies might include "think, pair, share" or "the muddiest point" which provides learners with space to reflect on challenging areas of the pre-work. Conversations can also be expanded by prompting learners with new example case studies to work through and apply new knowledge. Some examples of this approach have been published previously in the literature and showed improved learner familiarity and confidence with the topics discussed [37–43].
- Provide multiple podcast excerpts to different groups to provide a basis for a role-playing or jigsaw exercise. The "jigsaw" technique is a cooperative learning method where students become experts on a specific aspect of a topic and then teach their knowledge to their peers. Students may also be split into differing viewpoints or roles to discuss or debate varied perspectives on a topic. A debate type format to discuss a topic and compare approaches can promote critical thinking and lively discussions of evidence based medicine [44].
- Provide an instructional podcast or video that discusses the steps of a clinical procedure as prework, and use the synchronous session to practice a simulated procedure or case-based scenarios
- Learners can reflect on podcast material with exercises creating an infographic or concept map (individually or as a team), which allows the pairing of visual representations of relationships between concepts discussed in the podcast.
- Learners can consolidate their knowledge through polling or gamification type activities in the classroom, such as an audience response system or team-based quiz competition

For any activity, educators can consider a post-class phase as well where students have reflection activities, applications exercises, or assessments that reinforce learning and provide feedback. A podcast episode itself can also serve as that post-class activity, where learners listen as a follow-up on the concept.

Collaborate and Partner with Learners

While existing educational podcasts provide valuable resources, medical educators may encounter situations where pre-existing content fails to meet specific learning objectives or address unique educational needs. Details on creation of podcasts are outlined in previous chapters, but this section will highlight and explore the strategic integration of trainee-created podcast content as an innovative approach to medical education.

Educational Benefits of Trainee-Created Content

The process of creating podcast content represents a powerful pedagogical strategy that can take a learner from typical passive learning directly to creation of new material [45]. By engaging in the research and construction of an episode, trainees can transform their knowledge and enhance the understanding and retention of complex medical concepts. Participation in podcast creation can also augment a sense of community, introduce opportunities for mentorship, and facilitate professional identity formation [46]. Podcast creation also provides a deliberate practice activity for communication skill development. Depending on the level of involvement, technical skills acquisition is possible as well if students are involved in the production process, such as recording and editing.

Implementation Models

Trainees may choose to partner with pre-existing podcast platforms, which often welcome or recruit contributions to individual episodes or series of episodes [47–49]. Certain podcast platforms may have additional pathways to collaborate on a longitudinal basis. The benefit of partnering is that participation can focus on content creation and connecting with a larger community of practice, as the logistical framework for producing the podcast is already in place.

Educators can consider how to support and facilitate trainees in the creation of new materials as well, possibly with local or institutional support. This may include assisting in the needs assessment, design, and evaluation of a new project [50, 51]. Rotations in digital education or podcasting could be offered to support trainees who desire dedicated time to gain skills related to podcast creation and production. These rotations may be focused on social media or digital education, or alternatively integrated into pre-existing teaching curriculums [52]. Faculty mentorship would be critical to ensure a meaningful experience, and learners would benefit from structured frameworks and templates for content development if available.

Lastly, trainees and educators may also participate in various digital education training programs, which have been designed to equip healthcare professionals with the necessary tools, frameworks, and mentorship to create effective online resources, such as podcasts [52–60].

Continuing Medical Education (CME)

The audience of medical education podcasts extends beyond trainees and encompasses a broad spectrum of healthcare professionals. Many podcasts offer Continuing Medical Education (CME), Maintenance of Certification (MOC), or Continuing Education (CE) credits. A recent analysis in 2022 found that about 40% of podcasts intended for physician education provided CME offerings, and substantial use of CME has been demonstrated in various specialties including internal medicine, pediatrics, and emergency medicine [61–66].

Evaluation & Accreditation Process

CME/MOC/CE credits can be sponsored through individual programs via the appropriate accreditation councils, such as Accreditation Council for Continuing Medical Education (ACCME), the American Nurses Credentialing Center (ANCC), and the Accreditation Council for Pharmacy Education (ACPE). For example, the ACCME accredits organizations to provide CME for physicians. Organizations granted accreditation may include state medical societies, Liaison Committee for Medical Education (LCME)-accredited schools of medicine, or national physician membership organizations or specialty/subspecialty societies. While the ACCME provides accreditation, the individual organizations retain responsibility for designing, implementing, and reviewing the individual educational activities.

Podcast creators can request for CME credit from a relevant medical society or institution. This application process may vary slightly depending on organization, but key components typically required for CME credit of enduring materials like podcasts include:

- Podcast title and description
- Specific accreditation type(s) requested
- Clear objectives and anticipated learning outcomes
- Additional specifications may include:
  - Target professional audience (physicians, nurses, pharmacists/pharmacy technicians, physician assistants, etc.)
  - Identified professional or knowledge gap (including needs assessment results)
  - Content type: clinical, non-clinical (such as leadership, communication, ethics, or other professional topics), or both?
  - Learning approach: whether activity is knowledge-, application-, or practice-based
  - How the content is designed and reviewed
- Specific requirements for credit attainment, including minimum completion standard and assessment mechanisms

  - Example: listening to entire activity and successful completion of a post-test with a result of 75% or higher
- Administrative details: proposed activity duration, start and end dates, activity director and/or planning group information

Effective Implementation of Podcast-CME

Podcast-based CME must adhere to accreditation standards including evidence-based content with clear disclosure of any potential conflicts of interest. Explicit, measurable learning objectives should be used with each episode that align with practice needs. Participants should be provided easy to follow instructions on how to obtain CME credit, and CME systems will have an electronic method to assist in tracking completion and issuing credits.

Assessment mechanisms are often post-activity knowledge quizzes that can evaluate the retention and clinical application or practice impact surveys (of how podcast CME influenced clinical practice). Implementation models might include stand-alone CME episodes which are self-contained with an integrated assessment. Other strategies might include series-based credits (awarded upon completion of a topical series) or hybrid models (combining podcast content with live discussion or application activities).

Appropriately designed electronic CME has been demonstrated as equivalent to traditional face-to-face or live interactive CME sessions in measurements of immediate and sustained knowledge, self-reported behavior changes in practice, physician confidence, and use of evidence-based choices [67–71]. Offering CME can also improve the perceived credibility of digital resources [62, 65, 72]. Podcasts are an excellent educational tool that can be updated with relative ease to share timely clinical practice updates to a broad audience, and pairing this resource with CME delivery leverages an effective and economical way to disseminate knowledge when time or expense of travel limits access to more traditional CME activities.

References

1. Kelly JM, Perseghin A, Dow AW, Trivedi SP, Rodman A, Berk J. Learning through listening: a scoping review of podcast use in medical education. Acad Med J Assoc Am Med Coll. 2022;97(7):1079–85. https://doi.org/10.1097/ACM.0000000000004565.
2. Thomas PA, Kern DE, Hughes MT, Chen BY. Curriculum development for medical education: a six-step approach. JHU Press; 2016.
3. Woods JM, Chan TM, Roland D, Riddell J, Tagg A, Thoma B. Evaluating the reliability of gestalt quality ratings of medical education podcasts: a METRIQ study. Perspect Med Educ. 2020;9(5):302–6. https://doi.org/10.1007/s40037-020-00589-x.
4. Lin M, Thoma B, Trueger NS, Ankel F, Sherbino J, Chan T. Quality indicators for blogs and podcasts used in medical education: modified Delphi consensus recommendations by an

international cohort of health professions educators. Postgrad Med J. 2015;91(1080):546–50. https://doi.org/10.1136/postgradmedj-2014-133230.
5. Chan TMY, Grock A, Paddock M, Kulasegaram K, Yarris LM, Lin M. Examining reliability and validity of an online score (ALiEM AIR) for rating free open access medical education resources. Ann Emerg Med. 2016;68(6):729–35. https://doi.org/10.1016/j.annemergmed.2016.02.018.
6. Colmers-Gray IN, Krishnan K, Chan TM, et al. The revised METRIQ score: a quality evaluation tool for online educational resources. AEM Educ Train. 2019;3(4):387–92. https://doi.org/10.1002/aet2.10376.
7. Colmers I, Paterson Q, Lin M, Thoma B, Chan T. The quality checklists for medical education blogs and podcasts. The Winnower. Published online 2015. https://doi.org/10.15200/winn.144720.08769.
8. Lin M, Joshi N, Grock A, et al. Approved instructional resources series: a National Initiative to identify quality emergency medicine blog and podcast content for resident education. J Grad Med Educ. 2016;8(2):219–25. https://doi.org/10.4300/JGME-D-15-00388.1.
9. Paterson QS, Thoma B, Milne WK, Lin M, Chan TM. A systematic review and qualitative analysis to determine quality indicators for health professions education blogs and podcasts. J Grad Med Educ. 2015;7(4):549–54. https://doi.org/10.4300/JGME-D-14-00728.1.
10. Malecki SL, Quinn KL, Zilbert N, et al. Understanding the use and perceived impact of a medical podcast: qualitative study. JMIR Med Educ. 2019;5(2):e12901. https://doi.org/10.2196/12901.
11. Riddell J, Robins L, Brown A, Sherbino J, Lin M, Ilgen JS. Independent and interwoven: a qualitative exploration of residents' experiences with educational podcasts. Acad Med. 2020;95(1):89. https://doi.org/10.1097/ACM.0000000000002984.
12. Taylor DCM, Hamdy H. Adult learning theories: implications for learning and teaching in medical education: AMEE Guide No. 83. Med Teach. 2013;35(11):e1561–72. https://doi.org/10.3109/0142159X.2013.828153.
13. Mallin M, Schlein S, Doctor S, Stroud S, Dawson M, Fix M. A survey of the current utilization of asynchronous education among emergency medicine residents in the United States. Acad Med J Assoc Am Med Coll. 2014;89(4):598–601. doi:https://doi.org/10.1097/ACM.0000000000000170.
14. Bernstein E, Bhardwaj N, Pfoh ER, Yudelevich E. A nationwide survey of educational resource utilization and perception among internal medicine residents. J Gen Intern Med. 2021;36(6):1598–604. https://doi.org/10.1007/s11606-020-06441-6.
15. Young JQ, Van Merrienboer J, Durning S, Ten Cate O. Cognitive load theory: implications for medical education: AMEE Guide No. 86. Med Teach. 2014;36(5):371–84. https://doi.org/10.3109/0142159X.2014.889290.
16. Donald Boudreau J, Cassell, Eric, Fuks A. Preparing medical students to become attentive listeners. Med Teach. 2009;31(1):22–9. https://doi.org/10.1080/01421590802350776.
17. Nawaz Z, Mahboob U. Teaching attentive listening to medical students: need and strategies. J Pak Med Assoc. 2023;73(5):1076–8. https://doi.org/10.47391/JPMA.6023.
18. Coelho KR, Galan C. Physician cross-cultural nonverbal communication skills, patient satisfaction and health outcomes in the physician-patient relationship. Int J Fam Med. 2012;2012:376907. https://doi.org/10.1155/2012/376907.
19. Tennant K, Long A, Toney-Butler TJ. Active listening. In: StatPearls. StatPearls Publishing; 2025. Accessed 26 Mar 2025. http://www.ncbi.nlm.nih.gov/books/NBK442015/.
20. Weinstein Y, Sumeracki M, Caviglioli O. Understanding how we learn: a visual guide. Routledge; 2018.
21. Nebel C. Considerations for applying six strategies for effective learning to instruction. Med Sci Educ. 2020;30(Suppl 1):9–10. https://doi.org/10.1007/s40670-020-01088-8.
22. The Learning Scientists. The learning scientists. Accessed 26 Mar 2025. https://www.learningscientists.org
23. Madan CR. Using evidence-based learning strategies to improve medical education. Med Sci Educ. 2023;33(3):773–6. https://doi.org/10.1007/s40670-023-01798-9.

24. Benjamin AS, Tullis J. What makes distributed practice effective? Cognit Psychol. 2010;61(3):228–47. https://doi.org/10.1016/j.cogpsych.2010.05.004.
25. Cepeda NJ, Vul E, Rohrer D, Wixted JT, Pashler H. Spacing effects in learning: a temporal ridgeline of optimal retention. Psychol Sci. 2008;19(11):1095–102. https://doi.org/10.1111/j.1467-9280.2008.02209.x.
26. Using Spacing to Enhance Diverse Forms of Learning: Review of Recent Research and Implications for Instruction. Accessed 26 Mar 2025. https://www.researchgate.net/publication/235983059_Using_Spacing_to_Enhance_Diverse_Forms_of_Learning_Review_of_Recent_Research_and_Implications_for_Instruction
27. Van Hoof TJ, Sumeracki MA, Madan CR. Science of learning strategy series: article 3, interleaving. J Contin Educ Health Prof. 2022;42(4):265–8. https://doi.org/10.1097/CEH.0000000000000418.
28. The effects of interleaved practice—Taylor—2010—Applied Cognitive Psychology. Wiley Online Library. Accessed 26 Mar 2025. https://onlinelibrary.wiley.com/doi/abs/10.1002/acp.1598
29. Pressley M, Symons S, MA MD, Snyder BL, Turnure JE. Elaborative interrogation facilitates acquisition of confusing facts. J Educ Psychol. 1988;80(3):268–78. https://doi.org/10.1037/0022-0663.80.3.268.
30. Woloshyn VE, Pressley M, Schneider W. Elaborative-interrogation and prior-knowledge effects on learning of facts. J Educ Psychol. 1992;84(1):115–24. https://doi.org/10.1037/0022-0663.84.1.115.
31. Managing split-attention and redundancy in multimedia instruction. Accessed 26 Mar 2025. https://awspntest.apa.org/record/1999-03827-004
32. HEW KF, LO CK. Flipped classroom improves student learning in health professions education: a meta-analysis. BMC Med Educ. 2018;18(1):38. https://doi.org/10.1186/s12909-018-1144-z.
33. Hwang GJ, Chen PY. Effects of a collective problem-solving promotion-based flipped classroom on students' learning performances and interactive patterns. Interact Learn Environ. 2023;31(5):2513–28. https://doi.org/10.1080/10494820.2019.1568263.
34. Hurtubise L, Hall E, Sheridan L, Han H. The flipped classroom in medical education: engaging students to build competency. J Med Educat Curri Develop. 2015;2:JMECD.S23895. https://doi.org/10.4137/JMECD.S23895.
35. Schumacher DJ, Englander R, Carraccio C. Developing the master learner: applying learning theory to the learner, the teacher, and the learning environment. Acad Med J Assoc Am Med Coll. 2013;88(11):1635–45. https://doi.org/10.1097/ACM.0b013e3182a6e8f8.
36. Blair RA, Caton JB, Hamnvik OPR. A flipped classroom in graduate medical education. Clin Teach. 2020;17(2):195–9. https://doi.org/10.1111/tct.13091.
37. Ratliff JB, Nascimento FA, Tornes L, et al. Curriculum innovations: a podcast-based neurologic emergency flipped classroom curriculum for neurology residents. Neurol Educ. 2023;2(3):e200081. https://doi.org/10.1212/NE9.0000000000200081.
38. Lewis CE, Chen DC, Relan A. Implementation of a flipped classroom approach to promote active learning in the third-year surgery clerkship. Am J Surg. 2018;215(2):298–303. https://doi.org/10.1016/j.amjsurg.2017.08.050.
39. Coleman A, Lehman D. A flipped classroom and case-based curriculum to prepare medical students for vaccine-related conversations with parents. MedEdPORTAL. 2017;13:10582. https://doi.org/10.15766/mep_2374-8265.10582.
40. Moolchandani P, Chuang K, Larsen T. Patel S. VA GLA Medicine Podcast Club.
41. Mnatzaganian CL, Singh RF, Best BM, Morello CM. Effectiveness of providing video podcasts to pharmacy students in a self-study pharmaceutical calculations module. Am J Pharm Educ. 2020;84(12) https://doi.org/10.5688/ajpe7977.
42. Aljaber N, Alsaidan J, Shebl N, Almanasef M. Flipped classrooms in pharmacy education: a systematic review. Saudi Pharm J. 2023;31(12):101873. https://doi.org/10.1016/j.jsps.2023.101873.

43. Pham J, Tran A, O'Leary KS, Youm J, Tran DK, Chen JW. Neurosurgery lectures benefit from a flipped class approach. World Neurosurg. 2022;164:e481–91. https://doi.org/10.1016/j.wneu.2022.04.134.
44. Scott KR, Hsu CH, Johnson NJ, Mamtani M, Conlon LW, DeRoos FJ. Integration of social media in emergency medicine residency curriculum. Ann Emerg Med. 2014;64(4):396–404. https://doi.org/10.1016/j.annemergmed.2014.05.030.
45. Pangaro L, ten Cate O. Frameworks for learner assessment in medicine: AMEE Guide No. 78. Med Teach. 2013;35(6):e1197–210. https://doi.org/10.3109/0142159X.2013.788789.
46. Milligan KJ, Daulton RS, St Clair ZT, Epperson MV, Holloway RM, Schlaudecker JD. Creation of a student-run medical education podcast: tutorial. JMIR Med Educ. 2021;7(3):e29157. https://doi.org/10.2196/29157.
47. Merali Z, Carayannopoulos KL, Lai A. Exploring resident motivation with a podcast creation activity: a qualitative study. Med Sci Educ. 2023;33(6):1525–32. https://doi.org/10.1007/s40670-023-01921-w.
48. Ow GM, Shipley LC, Nematollahi S, Stetson GV. Morning report for all: a qualitative study of disseminating case conferences via podcasting. BMC Med Educ. 2021;21(1):392. https://doi.org/10.1186/s12909-021-02799-1.
49. Lau YTK, Alemán MJ, Medina R, Brondfield S, Nematollahi S. Around the world in 60 minutes: how a virtual morning report has created an International Community for Clinical Reasoning and Medical Education. Teach Learn Med. Published online June 21, 2023:1–10. https://doi.org/10.1080/10401334.2023.2226661.
50. Ghiathi C, Seitz K, Kritek P. How to create and evaluate a resident-led audio program: six clinical podcasts for medicine house staff. MedEdPORTAL. 16:11062. https://doi.org/10.15766/mep_2374-8265.11062.
51. Miller KA, Keeney T, Fialkowski A, et al. Leveraging podcasts to introduce medical students to the broader community of health care professionals. MedEdPORTAL. 17:11191. https://doi.org/10.15766/mep_2374-8265.11191.
52. Trivedi S, Saunders S, Rodman A. Strategies for designing a health professions digital education curriculum. Clin Teach. 2021;18(4):336–40. https://doi.org/10.1111/tct.13382.
53. Ramakrishnan M, Sparks MA, Farouk SS. Training the public physician: the nephrology social media collective internship. Semin Nephrol. 2020;40(3):320–7. https://doi.org/10.1016/j.semnephrol.2020.04.012.
54. Shah S, Topf J. Mentorship in the digital age: nephrology social media collective internship. Clin J Am Soc Nephrol. 2019;14(2):294–6. https://doi.org/10.2215/CJN.09970818.
55. Goyal A, Ambinder D, Farr M. Collab, virtualize, democratize: a conversation with the founders of CardioNerds. Circulation. 2022;146(4):269–75. https://doi.org/10.1161/CIRCULATIONAHA.122.061404.
56. Kotsenas AL, Aase L, Arce M, et al. The social media DNA of mayo clinic- and health care. J Am Coll Radiol. 2018;15(1 Pt B):162–6. https://doi.org/10.1016/j.jacr.2017.09.026.
57. Chan TM, Gottlieb M, Sherbino J, et al. The ALiEM faculty incubator: a novel online approach to faculty development in education scholarship. Acad Med J Assoc Am Med Coll. 2018;93(10):1497–502. https://doi.org/10.1097/ACM.0000000000002309.
58. Dong SW, Walker J, Nematollahi S, Nolan NS, Ryder JH. The ID digital institute: building a digital education toolset and community. Transplant Infect Dis. 2024;26(4):e14297. https://doi.org/10.1111/tid.14297.
59. Transforming your teaching using technology. Harvard Macy Institute. Accessed 24 Apr 2024. https://harvardmacy.org/courses/ttve
60. Surgery Education Fellowship. Behind the Knife About Us. Accessed 23 Apr 2024. https://behindtheknife.org/about
61. Zhang E, Trad N, Corty R, Zohrob D, Trivedi S, Rodman A. How podcasts teach: a comprehensive analysis of the didactic methods of the top hundred medical podcasts. Med Teach. 2022;44(10):1146–50. https://doi.org/10.1080/0142159X.2022.2071691.

62. Patrick MD, Stukus DR, Nuss KE. Using podcasts to deliver pediatric educational content: development and reach of PediaCast CME. Digit Health. 2019;5:2055207619834842. https://doi.org/10.1177/2055207619834842.
63. Berk J, Trivedi SP, Watto M, Williams P, Centor R. Medical education podcasts: where we are and questions unanswered. J Gen Intern Med. 2020;35(7):2176–8. https://doi.org/10.1007/s11606-019-05606-2.
64. Tarchichi TR, Szymusiak J. Continuing medical education in the time of social distancing: the case for expanding podcast usage for continuing education. J Contin Educ Heal Prof. 2021;41(1):70–4. https://doi.org/10.1097/CEH.0000000000000324.
65. Young KJ, Kim JJ, Yeung G, Sit C, Tobe SW. Physician preferences for accredited online continuing medical education. J Contin Educ Heal Prof. 2011;31(4):241–6. https://doi.org/10.1002/chp.20136.
66. Kelly JM, Perseghin A, Dow A, et al. Continuing education evaluations of an internal medicine and a pediatric podcast. J Contin Educ Heal Prof. 2023;43(4):283. https://doi.org/10.1097/CEH.0000000000000501.
67. Fordis M, King JE, Ballantyne CM, et al. Comparison of the instructional efficacy of Internet-based CME with live interactive CME workshops: a randomized controlled trial. JAMA. 2005;294(9):1043–51. https://doi.org/10.1001/jama.294.9.1043.
68. Curran V, Lockyer J, Sargeant J, Fleet L. Evaluation of learning outcomes in Web-based continuing medical education. Acad Med J Assoc Am Med Coll. 2006;81(10 Suppl):S30–4. https://doi.org/10.1097/01.ACM.0000236509.32699.f5.
69. Curran VR, Fleet LJ, Kirby F. A comparative evaluation of the effect of Internet-based CME delivery format on satisfaction, knowledge and confidence. BMC Med Educ. 2010;10:10. https://doi.org/10.1186/1472-6920-10-10.
70. Casebeer L, Brown J, Roepke N, et al. Evidence-based choices of physicians: a comparative analysis of physicians participating in Internet CME and non-participants. BMC Med Educ. 2010;10:42. https://doi.org/10.1186/1472-6920-10-42.
71. Cook DA, Levinson AJ, Garside S, Dupras DM, Erwin PJ, Montori VM. Internet-based learning in the health professions: a meta-analysis. JAMA. 2008;300(10):1181–96. https://doi.org/10.1001/jama.300.10.1181.
72. Harris JM, Sklar BM, Amend RW, Novalis-Marine C. The growth, characteristics, and future of online CME. J Contin Educ Heal Prof. 2010;30(1):3–10. https://doi.org/10.1002/chp.20050.

Chapter 13
Health Equity and Podcasting

Angela Castellanos and Edith Bracho-Sanchez

Health Equity and Health Disparities in Health Information

Despite national public health initiatives and institutional commitments to reducing health disparities in the United States, people who don't speak English as a primary language, who live in rural areas, who come from communities underserved by the medical system, or from communities that experience structural and overt racism, have worse health outcomes than those who belong to the socio-cultural majority in the US. Studies have demonstrated that hospitalized children of families who speak languages other than English have more adverse health events than their English-speaking counterparts [16]; Black infants are more likely to die from Sudden Unexpected Infant Death than non-Hispanic white infants [32]; Rural communities have higher rates of cardiovascular disease [17] and Type 2 Diabetes [41]. Health disparities are defined by the Centers for Disease Control and Prevention as preventable differences that populations experience in the burden of disease, injury, violence, or opportunities. Health equity is, in turn, defined by the CDC as the state in which everyone has a fair and just opportunity to attain their highest level of health. The reasons behind these health disparities are complex and rooted in social determinants of health—people's work and home environment, education, economic stability and social, cultural, and community context, as well as structural bias and racism [37]. Additionally, differences in health literacy and in how communities interact with health information contribute to each of these disparities in the context

A. Castellanos (✉)
Division of Hospital Medicine, Department of Pediatrics, Stanford University School of Medicine, Stanford, CA, USA
e-mail: acastell@stanford.edu

E. Bracho-Sanchez
Division of Child and Adolescent Health, Department of Pediatrics, Columbia University Irving Medical Center, New York, NY, USA

J. Parga-Belinkie et al. (eds.), *Podcasting for Medical Professionals*,
https://doi.org/10.1007/978-3-032-16480-3_13

of social determinants of health: non-English speaking families who cannot read English-language medication labels, clinical notes, or results while in the hospital; ineffective public health messaging regarding Sudden Unexpected Infant Death risk factors in Black communities; lack of high-speed internet access in rural areas making it difficult to access cardiovascular and diabetes prevention information. Public health organizations, health institutions, and health content creators are turning toward health information outlets like podcasts to provide timely, accurate health information and improve health outcomes, so it is essential to keep health equity and the elimination of health disparities in mind when creating and disseminating this information.

Existing health information reaches communities in various ways, and communities have differences in preferred consumption habits. If unaccounted for in content creation, these preferences can leave the door open for health disparities in communication. For example, a 2011 study investigating cancer information-seeking behavior differences among people by race, ethnicity, language, and social class found that Spanish-speaking Hispanic participants were more likely to pay attention to and trust health information from the radio, while non-Hispanic Black participants were more likely to pay attention to and trust health information from television. The same study also found that college graduates were more likely to pay attention to health messages from print media and the internet than those who were not high school graduates [44]. Among adults who smoke in the US—an important group to consider when thinking about targeted public health messaging—access to high-speed internet is strongly associated with online health information seeking, and yet digital device ownership, high-speed internet access, and online health information seeking varies widely among non-Hispanic Black or African American adults and those with lower income and education levels [20]. Recognizing that the same podcast episode, public health message, or health information website may reach and be received differently by various communities in the US and abroad is vital to content creators when approaching their podcasts with a health equity lens.

Several marketing and research studies have demonstrated the emerging and evolving demographics of podcast listeners in the US as the medium increases in popularity. According to the Pew Research Center, podcast listeners are usually between the ages of 18 and 29 [15]. In a cross-sectional study that looked at the race and ethnicity of US listeners in the prior 12 months, the percentage of adults who had listened to at least one podcast was roughly similar across white (47%), black (46%), Hispanic (54%) and English-speaking Asian adults (52%) surveyed [33]. Another poll by Statistica demonstrates that while in 2018, most podcast listeners were college-educated, by 2024, the proportions of college-educated and non-college-educated were about even at 49% and 51%, respectively [13]. A 2019 study surveying caregivers and health care professionals at a pediatric primary care practice about podcast listening habits found that more than half of podcast-listening parents/caregivers had a bachelor's degree or higher. As a whole, podcast listeners were more likely to have higher incomes [18].

If creators are fortunate enough to have their content reach the ears of their selected listeners, how people receive and absorb this health information presents another opportunity for creators to consider differences in health literacy among different groups. Health literacy, defined by the US Department of Health and Human Services as the ability to find, understand, and use health information, is emerging as a key recognized factor in social determinants of health [12]. Research suggests that health literacy is likely a mediator of racial and socioeconomic health disparities. Low health literacy limits the ability to use health information to improve one's health and to access health services. Studies have shown that the prevalence of low health literacy can be as high as 70% in pediatric emergency rooms; low health literacy is also associated with limited injury prevention knowledge in caregivers, suboptimal parental feeding and nutrition behaviors for their children, and a predictor for tobacco use in adolescents. Low health literacy is more likely to be associated with racial and ethnic minorities, individuals with lower income or education attainment, and individuals who primarily speak languages other than English [23].

As the world becomes more reliant on digital technology, the concept of digital health literacy adds another layer of complexity for people navigating the health information landscape. The World Health Organization defines digital health literacy as "the ability to search, find, understand and evaluate health information from electronic resources and to use the knowledge gained to solve health-related problems [38]." While it may appear that digital health literacy is simply health literacy in a digital context, the reality is more complicated. For example, a person capable of reading a nutrition label to make an informed dietary choice may have difficulty selecting, downloading, and incorporating a nutrition tracking app into their life. While digital health literacy is an emerging field of research, literature reviews on the topic have reported that the characteristics of communities who historically experience health outcome disparities (non-white, rural, and lower income individuals) unsurprisingly overlap with those who face challenges with digital health tools [42].

Techquity and a Cautionary Telehealth Tale

If health equity can be defined as attaining the highest level of health for all by addressing avoidable health inequities and ensuring fair and just access [10], then what is *Techquity? Techquity*, a concept that emerged in the late 2010s, is defined by Rhee et al. as "the strategic development and deployment of technology in health care and health to achieve health equity" [27]. Digital connectivity and digital health literacy have been called "super" social determinants of health because of how interconnected the digital world is with all other social determinants of health [35] (Fig. 13.1).

According to the National Digital Inclusion Alliance, participation in the digital world requires (1) affordable broadband internet service, (2) Internet-enabled devices, (3) access to digital literacy training, (4) quality technical support, and (5) applications and online content designed to enable and encourage self-sufficiency,

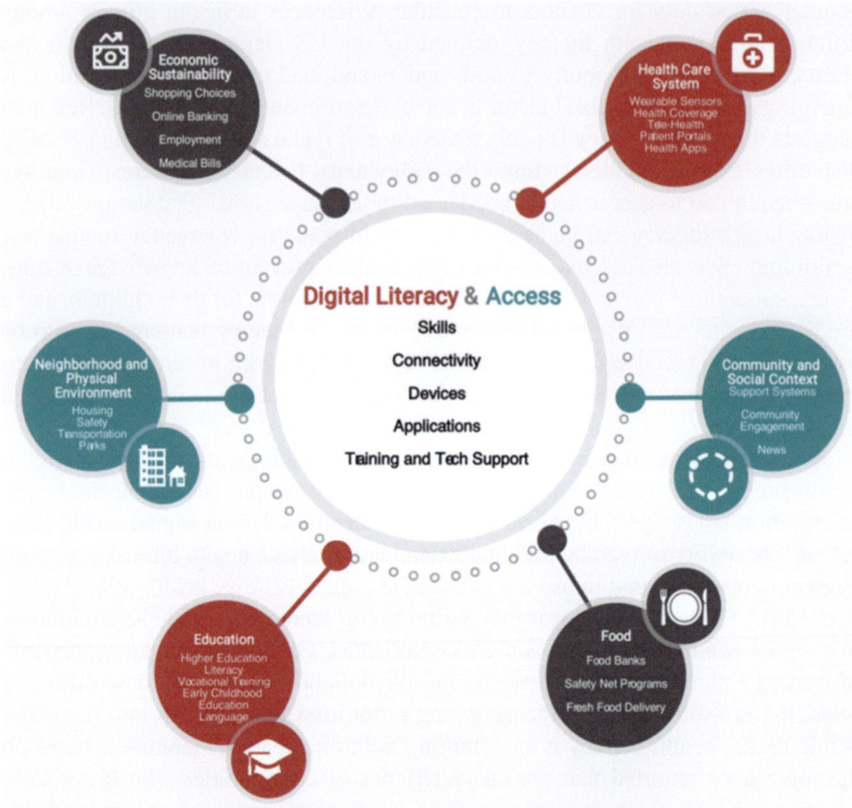

Fig. 13.1 Digital literacy and access, including skills, connectivity, devices and training and technical support, relate to all other domains of social determinants of health. (Sieck et al. [35])

participation, and collaboration [5]. *Techquity* can pertain to a variety of digital health tools, such as online health portals, health trackers and wearables, and artificial intelligence. We consider health information and communication through podcasting as an emerging digital health communication technology. Just as with any innovation, content creators must be mindful of the limitations of digital connectivity and digital health literacy in reaching their audience. The emergence and adoption of telehealth in the late 2010s and early 2020s serves as a case study for how a technology that promised to overcome barriers was shown to perpetuate existing barriers and highlight new health inequities in some cases.

Telehealth is an important digital technology that holds promise in addressing health disparities in care access. Its wide adoption has shown the importance of "digital inclusion" as a social determinant of health. While telehealth showed promise in the late 2010s, its significance and utilization skyrocketed in 2020 with the COVID-19 pandemic. Although the pandemic kept all but the sickest patients home and away from medical care, patients continued to have needs related to serious chronic health conditions, mental health conditions, less acute medical problems, and disease prevention and surveillance. Without access to their healthcare providers, these needs went unmet unless telehealth was available. Less than one fourth of one percent of January 2020 medical claims were for provider-to-patient telehealth services [8]. That number increased to 13% in April 2020 and settled around 4% in 2021 [8]. As demand grew, health systems saw telehealth as a viable and equitable solution—not only would telehealth support patient visits during the pandemic, but now patients who lived hours from the clinic, lacked reliable transportation, or had difficulties navigating the physical world could still make their appointments. All patients and doctors had to do was log on.

In practice, however, telehealth was not always the silver bullet it promised to be; in fact, it highlighted barriers to access that perpetuated health disparities. One study of cancer patients in the University of California San Diego Health System demonstrated that among the almost 30% of nearly 30,000 patient encounters in 2020 conducted via telemedicine, several groups were significantly less likely to use the service, including Hispanic, Spanish-speaking, Asian and low-income patients [26]. Patients in rural areas have also historically had limited access to broadband internet to facilitate virtual visits. While phones are an option, one report states that while 95% of US rural residents own a cellphone, just 71% own a smartphone, restricting access to telehealth services to those who have the appropriate video capabilities [6].

Telemedicine, as equitable as it may seem, relies on a stable technical infrastructure, language concordance or interpretation access, digital literacy, private space, and readily available technical support. Challenges in any of these domains render the technology inaccessible. Yet, when planned and implemented with a health equity lens, telehealth can fulfill its promise of expanding access to care. A 2024 study by Pathak et al. examined telemedicine access and utilization within a pediatric, low-income, primarily Latino population. The study found that, despite socioeconomic challenges, families were able to engage with telehealth services effectively when provided with appropriate support and resources. This underscores that disparities in access are preventable. With intentional design, inclusive infrastructure, and continuous evaluation, telehealth can serve as a vehicle for equity rather than exacerbating existing gaps [25].

Podcasting shows much of the same promise for lowering barriers to health information as telemedicine does for providing access to care. Like telemedicine, podcasts are typically free for listeners, available via the internet, and accessible via smartphones. Like telemedicine, podcasts require access to the internet, language concordance, and a reasonable degree of digital and health literacy. Unlike telemedicine, however, podcasts do not typically come directly from a healthcare provider invested in the patient's health, helping to troubleshoot if a patient cannot log on. Podcasts require their listeners to find the content, download the apps, appraise the creators and their content, and distinguish between opinion and fact. As content creators, we can support our listeners by intentionally creating and disseminating content that centers health equity and minimizes bias. A variety of frameworks have been proposed to consider health equity when creating and implementing digital health technologies. Here, we review an approach and propose an adapted framework to help podcast producers approach content creation and dissemination with a health equity lens.

Ensuring Digital Health Equity for Podcast Consumers—Existing Frameworks for Creator Consideration

As healthcare providers, when we provide health information or create public content, we risk creating from our own biased perspective. We have expert-level medical knowledge; we constantly speak and think about disease, illness, and prevention in our own professional jargon and review statistics that, without context, are too abstract to ground decision-making for the average listener. An effective health communicator serves as an interpreter of this information, but we must also be cognizant that our tools for dissemination are subject to these biases. Frameworks and protocols help counteract these biases by offering a structured, evidence-informed process that prompts creators to consider equity, context, and audience at each stage of design and dissemination. There is a growing body of work describing implementation frameworks to specifically center health equity in healthcare interventions [7, 24, 45]. With the growth of digital health technologies, researchers and practitioners are developing frameworks especially for this domain. For example, the "Framework for Digital Health Equity" creates an expansion of the leading health disparities framework from the National Institute on Minority Health and Health Disparities, adding "the digital environment" as a domain of influence and the levels of influence at the individual, interpersonal, community and societal level [28] (Fig. 13.2). We will use this approach to discuss how podcasts are embedded in the social determinants of health and how podcast creators can consider these determinants when creating and disseminating their podcasts.

Applying the NIMHHD Framework to Podcasting with a Health Equity Lens

Level of Influence: Individual

In the digital environment, the relationship between the podcaster and the individual is at the core of the medium. Thus, content creators must consider the individual needs of audience members to engage with their content.

Questions to consider for podcasters:

- How digitally literate is the intended listener?
- What is the health literacy level of the intended listener?

Domains of Influence (Over the Lifecourse)	Levels of Influence*			
	Individual	Interpersonal	Community	Societal
Biological	Biological Vulnerability and Mechanisms	Caregiver–Child Interaction Family Microbiome	Community Illness Exposure Herd Immunity	Sanitation Immunization Pathogen Exposure
Behavioral	Health Behaviors Coping Strategies	Family Functioning School/Work Functioning	Community Functioning	Policies and Laws
Physical/Built Environment	Personal Environment	Household Environment School/Work Environment	Community Environment Community Resources	Societal Structure
Digital Environment	Digital Literacy, Digital Self-Efficacy, Technology Access, Attitudes Towards Use	Implicit Tech Bias, Interdependence (e.g. shared devices), Patient-Tech-Clinician Relationship	Community Infrastructure, Healthcare Infrastructure, Community Tech Norms, Community Partners	Tech Policy, Data Standards, Design Standards, Social Norms & Ideologies, Algorithmic Bias
Sociocultural Environment	Sociodemographics Limited English Cultural Identity Response to Discrimination	Social Networks Family/Peer Norms Interpersonal Discrimination	Community Norms Local Structural Discrimination	Social Norms Societal Structural Discrimination
Health Care System	Insurance Coverage Health Literacy Treatment Preferences	Patient–Clinician Relationship Medical Decision-Making	Availability of Services Safety Net Services	Quality of Care Health Care Policies
Health Outcomes	Individual Health	Family/ Organizational Health	Community Health	Population Health

Fig. 13.2 National Institute on Minority Health and Health Disparities Research Framework Expanded for Digital Health Equity (Richardson et al. [28])

- Does the intended listener have access to the Internet, computer, or smartphone to listen to the podcast? Can they download the appropriate application? How can we mitigate this digital health literacy barrier?
- Can the intended listener effectively and effortlessly use the podcasting platform (Digital Self-efficacy)?
- Does the community you wish to engage frequently use podcasts and trust digital health information?

Level of Influence: Interpersonal

- What are the creator's implicit tech biases of the podcast's intended population?
- Is there interdependence of devices in the community, and if so, how does that affect podcast usage?
- Patient-Tech-Clinician relationship: In the case of podcasting, this can be thought of as the Listener-Tech-Creator relationship. Podcasts may allow for ease of access to health information and introduction to other health information podcasts, opening conversations between health care providers and patients about their health and any other related stigmatized or rarely addressed but important topics.

Level of Influence: Community

- What is internet access like in the community? Is it affordable? Does downloading and listening to the podcast require a high-quality internet connection?
- How are you marketing your podcast? How does the community engage on social media, and on what platforms? Where can you reach community members directly to introduce them to your podcast? Can you partner with a community organization to develop a trusting, mutually beneficial, and educational relationship with listeners?

Level of Influence: Societal

- What are the policies that affect a listener's ability to access podcasts? Is there access to broadband networks?
- When marketing your podcast, are there algorithmic biases or policies that would impede your ability to connect with your desired audience?
- Are social norms around topics or populations impeding your ability to connect with your audience? How can you overcome those?

Podcasts as Tools for Advancing Health Equity

At their core, health information podcasts are public health efforts. Podcasting can bolster a systems approach to public health problems by providing another avenue to advance health literacy and people's ability to find, understand, and use health information. Podcasting can address social inequities through a variety of ways—by providing accessible, timely health education information produced by medical experts, institutions and publications; by overcoming barriers of time and space; by connecting people across languages and experiences, and by humanizing health issues related to immigration, gender, racism and sexual orientation.

Current Examples of Podcasts Addressing Health Disparities

Improving Health Information Accessibility Through Podcasting

1. **Making health education more widely available and affordable**

In a 2024 Nature Medicine Correspondence, van Niekerk et al. wrote: "Podcasts have emerged as a powerful and accessible communication platform that holds promise for its ability to challenge knowledge silos, hierarchies and incentive structures in public health…" citing the podcasts' ability to cross hierarchies, institutions, and disciplines "without being constrained by geographic, cultural or financial barriers" [43]. Health education and medical literature were once limited to textbooks, medical school classrooms, and subscription-based peer-reviewed medical journals. With podcasting, preeminent medical journals, such as the New England Journal of Medicine, and public health institutions, such as Johns Hopkins University, share their latest research and innovations via free podcasts with the world. Since 2020, The American Academy of Pediatrics has published podcasts for parents and practitioners, disseminating their latest guideline updates and providing free, timely health information that was once kept behind a paywall. OPENPediatrics, supported by Boston Children's Hospital, requires only a free log-in for access to pediatric medical education podcasts with the express purpose of providing accessible medical education content for resource-limited healthcare providers worldwide. Collectively, these developments underscore podcasting's growing role in medical and public health communication, enabling the widespread dissemination of evidence-based knowledge beyond traditional academic and institutional boundaries.

2. **Sharing information and connection across boundaries of time and space**

Health providers with communication expertise who appear on local news or at health fairs help disseminate health information to communities, but only to those who can tune in or make it to the event. Often, those who are at the highest risk of health disparities are those who work long shifts, work on the weekends, and struggle to make it to their own doctor's appointments. Because podcasts are available on-demand, listeners can engage with them at their convenience, picking a time to maximize their engagement rather than relying on a network or health fair schedule. This on-demand nature also benefits those geographically isolated from trusted health information sources.

Health professionals from all over the world, both in academic and private settings, are using podcasting's on-demand and boundary-jumping reach to expand the reach of health information and advocacy. In India, the SMAART Lab, led by public health expert and scholar Dr. Ashish Joshi, created the SANGYAN podcast with episodes in multiple languages to address health misinformation in rural and urban Chennai, Tamil Nadu, India. They plan to study the health literacy and demographics of their listeners and the usability, acceptance, and user satisfaction of the podcast [14]. Similar to OPENPediatrics from Boston Children's Hospital, the Children's Hospital of Philadelphia Online Pediatrics Education Network (CHOP OPEN) from the institution's department of Global Pediatric Education, provides free online virtual courses and podcasts, sharing peer-reviewed medical educational content for healthcare professionals worldwide. Podcasts like The American Hospital Association's Rural Podcast Series spotlight and amplify challenges unique to rural hospitals, such as suicide prevention and behavioral health, cybersecurity, and employee retention in rural hospitals [1]. Dr. Randy Lehman hosts Rural American Surgeon, a podcast dedicated to sharing techniques and stories from rural operating rooms in the US and creating a community in an otherwise geographically isolating field that centers medically underserved patient populations [40].

3. **Fostering language access and cultural connection**

According to the US Census, about one out of five Americans speak languages other than English at home, the most common being Spanish, Chinese (including all dialects), and Tagalog [4]. Since patients who primarily speak languages other than English are more likely to have worse health outcomes, hospitals, universities, public health, and federal institutions must offer trusted health information in a variety of languages [16]. Health information delivered via podcast can help overcome written literacy issues and gives podcast producers an opportunity to engage experts and members of a specific community who not only speak the language but also act as cultural brokers to inspire trust with listeners. Programs such as JUNTOS Radio, from the JUNTOS Center for Advancing Latino Health at the University of Kansas Medical Center, produce podcast episodes on health topics relevant to the Latino community and highlight Spanish-speaking health professionals and members of the Latino community sharing health-related stories and resources [19]. The American Journal of Public Health publishes its podcast in English and Chinese, with its associate editor, Jihong Liu, serving as the Chinese-language host [2]. These efforts highlight the critical role multilingual podcasting can play in advancing linguistic equity in health communication, fostering trust, and improving health outcomes among linguistically diverse communities.

4. **Amplifying marginalized voices and stories**

Studies have demonstrated that language and race-concordant care improves patient outcomes and improves trust between patients and healthcare providers [11, 21, 22, 34, 36], so what if this approach can be applied to health information? While we can translate health information pamphlets, podcasts can connect with patients in ways that written information simply cannot. In podcasting, listeners can identify with and develop relationships with the hosts and guests, making the selection of the hosts and guests important, particularly if the podcast has topics and content aimed at underrepresented or marginalized communities or is exploring a nuanced subject such as immigration or racism. Podcasts offer greater opportunities for the inclusivity of voices, cultures, and perspectives. Authenticity in representation is imperative for podcast creators hoping to connect with underserved, underrepresented, or marginalized communities.

A few popular podcasts and media outlets have used their platform to elevate communities of color and highlight nuanced health equity topics on their podcasts. The Nocturnists, an award-winning medical storytelling podcast created a "Black Voices in Healthcare" series, hosted by physician Dr. Ashley McMullen and executive producer Dr. Kimberly Manning. More than 200 Black healthcare providers from across the US participated in the 10-episode series produced in 2020 in the wake of the murder of George Floyd. The series highlighted stories of racism in healthcare and also highlighted stories of "Black joy, Black love and Black excellence" and was a 2021 Webby Award honoree [3]. Popular internal medicine and pediatrics medical education podcast "The Curbsiders" uses their platform to take deeper dives into racism in medical practice and education and promote anti-racism, with episodes such as "Racism and Inequities in Addiction Medicine with Dr. Myra Mathis" or "Race Corrections in UTI Guidelines," featuring discussions with experts in health equity and clinical care and providing definitions, context and a safe space for learning about these nuanced topics for their listeners [39]. In 2022, WGBH, Boston's public radio station, teamed up with Harvard Medical School and *El Planeta*, a Spanish-language New England-based newspaper to produce *Salud*, a podcast produced in both English and Spanish that highlights timely health topics important to the Hispanic and Latino/a/x community and features health experts as well as the people facing these health challenges, such as a Mexican actor awaiting a lung transplant, a survivor of a fentanyl overdose and an immigrant who has lived in the US for 20 years who lost their health insurance [29]. In 2022, *Salud* reached more than 9000 listeners and had over more than 16,000 downloads [30].

Time and again, we have seen that stories and anecdotes connect with people better than facts and statistics, and podcasts offer a compelling format to highlight and illustrate nuanced topics with impactful stories supported by compelling, high-quality evidence. More podcast producers need to share data related to podcast reach, including listens and downloads, to better understand the impact of this content and facilitate the study of the podcast's effects on health education, trust, health information and health equity.

5. **Improving health literacy through podcasting**

Earlier in this chapter, we discussed the importance of considering health and digital literacy when creating podcasts. But what if podcasts could be used to improve health literacy as well? A few studies have shown promise in using podcasts as educational tools to empower patients to understand their health. A 2024 qualitative study using a podcast to prepare patients for hospital visits identified "enhanced engagement and empowerment through podcasts" among their participants [9]. A 2017 study published in *The Lancet* demonstrated a podcast that aimed to improve the ability of listeners in Uganda to assess claims about the risks and benefits of medical treatments and make informed health choices successfully improved knowledge around this topic compared to a public service announcement [31]. In the current social media climate of conflicting health recommendations and misinformation, more reputable, high-quality podcasts should aim to support listeners' abilities to wade through online information and identify appropriate, actionable, trustworthy, and reliable health information sources.

As demonstrated in the examples above, medical information podcast creators are working to center health equity by reducing barriers such as economic resources, health literacy, geographic isolation and language access, to high-quality health information.

Conclusion

Podcasting holds immense promise as a tool for health equity. It can cross borders of geography, culture, language, and institutional hierarchy to share lifesaving, empowering information directly with the people who need it most. But as with any digital health innovation, the potential to do good is accompanied by the risk of deepening existing disparities. Just as we have seen with telehealth, technology alone is not inherently equitable; equity must be built into its design, dissemination, and evaluation.

This chapter highlights how podcasting can advance health equity by making health education more accessible, amplifying marginalized voices, increasing language access, and offering connections across time and space. However, we've also underscored that podcast creators must approach this work intentionally — considering who their audience is, how they access and understand information, and whether their content truly reflects the needs and experiences of the communities they aim to serve.

Applying health equity frameworks such as the NIMHHD Digital Health Equity model offers podcast creators a structured way to interrogate their own biases, build trust with their audiences, and evaluate the impact of their work. These tools guide content creation and shape how we think about access in the digital public health space.

In a world where misinformation spreads rapidly, and health inequities persist, the opportunity—and responsibility—for podcasting as a health communication tool is clear. Podcasting alone cannot solve health disparities, but when wielded with care, intention, and community partnership, it can be part of a broader, transformative movement toward health justice.

As podcast creators, public health professionals, educators, and institutions, we must inform and examine the systems perpetuating exclusion. The next wave of health communication must not only speak louder—it must speak more equitably.

References

1. AHA's Rural Podcast Series | AHA. (n.d.). Retrieved April 7, 2025, from https://www.aha.org/advocacy/small-or-rural/rural-report-podcast-series
2. AJPH. (n.d.). Am J Public Health Retrieved April 7, 2025, from http://ajph.aphapublications.org/
3. Black Voices In Healthcare: The Nocturnists Podcast. (n.d.). Retrieved April 21, 2025, from https://thenocturnists.org/blackvoicesinhealthcare
4. Bureau, U. C. (n.d.) Nearly 68 million people spoke a language other than English at home in 2019. Census.Gov. Retrieved April 7, 2025, from https://www.census.gov/library/stories/2022/12/languages-we-speak-in-united-states.html
5. Definitions. (n.d.). National digital inclusion alliance. Retrieved March 20, 2025, from https://dev.digitalinclusion.org/definitions/

6. DeGuzman PB, Siegfried Z, Leimkuhler ME. Evaluation of rural public libraries to address telemedicine inequities. Public Health Nurs. 2020;37(5):806–11. https://doi.org/10.1111/phn.12777.
7. Eslava-Schmalbach J, Garzón-Orjuela N, Elias V, Reveiz L, Tran N, Langlois EV. Conceptual framework of equity-focused implementation research for health programs (EquIR). Int J Equity Health. 2019;18(1):80. https://doi.org/10.1186/s12939-019-0984-4.
8. Edmiston KD, AlZuBi J. Trends in telehealth and its implications for health disparities (Center for Insurance Policy & Research Report). National Association of Insurance Commissioners. 2022. https://content.naic.org/sites/default/files/Telehealth%20and%20Health%20Disparities.pdf.
9. Frølund JC, Løkke A, Jensen HI, Farver-Vestergaard I. The use of podcasts as Patient preparation for hospital visits—an interview study exploring patients' experiences. Int J Environ Res Public Health. 2024;21(6):746. https://doi.org/10.3390/ijerph21060746.
10. Gómez CA, Kleinman DV, Pronk N, Wrenn Gordon GL, Ochiai E, Blakey C, Johnson A, Brewer KH. Addressing health equity and social determinants of health through healthy people 2030. J Public Health Manag Pract. 2021;27(6):S249–57. https://doi.org/10.1097/PHH.0000000000001297.
11. Greenwood BN, Hardeman RR, Huang L, Sojourner A. Physician–patient racial concordance and disparities in birthing mortality for newborns. Proc Natl Acad Sci USA. 2020;117(35):21194–200. https://doi.org/10.1073/pnas.1913405117.
12. Health Literacy in Healthy People 2030—Healthy People 2030 | odphp.health.gov. (n.d.). Retrieved April 7, 2025, from https://odphp.health.gov/healthypeople/priority-areas/health-literacy-healthy-people-2030
13. Infographic: Podcast Listeners Grow More Diverse. (2024, October 4). Statista Daily Data. https://www.statista.com/chart/15609/podcast-audience-characteristics
14. Joshi A, Mohan SK, Pandya AK, Grover A, Saggu SR, Revathi SK, Sharma S. Digital Health Intervention (SANGYAN podcast) to enhance knowledge related to COVID-19 and other Health conditions: protocol for an implementation and evaluation study. JMIR Research Protocols. 2025;14:e41175. https://doi.org/10.2196/41175.
15. Jurkowitz ES, Liedke J, Matsa KE, Mark ML (2023, April 18). 4. Podcast use among different age groups. Pew Research Center. https://www.pewresearch.org/journalism/2023/04/18/podcast-use-among-different-age-groups/
16. Khan A, Yin HS, Brach C, Graham DA, Ramotar MW, Williams DN, Spector N, Landrigan CP, Dreyer BP, Patient and family centered I-PASS health literacy subcommittee. Association between parent comfort with English and adverse events among hospitalized children. JAMA Pediatr. 2020;174(12):e203215. https://doi.org/10.1001/jamapediatrics.2020.3215.
17. Kulshreshtha A, Goyal A, Dabhadkar K, Veledar E, Vaccarino V. Urban-rural differences in coronary heart disease mortality in the United States: 1999–2009. Public Health Rep. 2014;129(1):19–29.
18. Lee C, Zhou MS, Wang ER, Huber M, Lockwood KK, Parga J. Health care professional and caregiver attitudes toward and usage of medical podcasting: questionnaire study. JMIR Pediatr Parent. 2022;5(1):e29857. https://doi.org/10.2196/29857.
19. Linares BM, Ramirez M. JUNTOS radio: a podcast created in collaboration with Spanish-speaking healthcare providers, Juntos Center for Advancing Latino Health, and a medical librarian. JMLA. 2023;111(4):831–2. https://doi.org/10.5195/jmla.2023.1653.
20. Long SE, D'Angelo H, Lama Y. Digital communication inequalities among U.S. adults reporting current cigarette use. Am J Prev Med. 2024;66(2):307–14. https://doi.org/10.1016/j.amepre.2023.09.025.
21. Luercio M, Quiñones-Pérez B, Castellanos A, Ngo T, Elder B, Blaine K, Haskell H, Lopez K, Luff D, Mallick N, Mercer AN, Williams DN, Baird JD, Khan A. Communicating with Spanish-speaking families of hospitalized children with medical complexity. Hosp Pediatr. 2024;14(8):612–21. https://doi.org/10.1542/hpeds.2023-007700.

22. Molina RL, Bazan M, Hacker MR, Kaimal AJ, Alegría M, Fernández L, Guise J-M, Edelen MO. A Spanish-language Patient-reported outcome measure for trust in pregnancy care clinician. JAMA Netw Open. 2025;8(2):e2460465. https://doi.org/10.1001/jamanetworkopen.2024.60465.
23. Morrison AK, Glick A, Yin HS. Health literacy: implications for child health. Pediatr Rev. 2019;40(6):263–77. https://doi.org/10.1542/pir.2018-0027.
24. Nápoles AM, Stewart AL. Transcreation: an implementation science framework for community-engaged behavioral interventions to reduce health disparities. BMC Health Serv Res. 2018;18:710. https://doi.org/10.1186/s12913-018-3521-z.
25. Pathak PR, Stockwell MS, Lane MM, Robbins-Milne L, Friedman S, Pethe K, Krause MC, Soren K, Matiz LA, Solomon LB, Burke ME, Bracho-Sanchez E. Access to primary care telemedicine and visit characterization in a pediatric, low-income, primarily Latino population: retrospective study. JMIR Pediatr Parent. 2024;7:e57702. https://doi.org/10.2196/57702.
26. Qian AS, Schiaffino MK, Nalawade V, Aziz L, Pacheco FV, Nguyen B, Vu P, Patel SP, Martinez ME, Murphy JD. Disparities in telemedicine during COVID-19. Cancer Med. 2022;11(4):1192–201. https://doi.org/10.1002/cam4.4518.
27. Rhee K, Dankwa-Mullan I, Brennan V, Clark C. What is TechQuity? J Health Care Poor Underserved. 2021;32(2):xiii–xviii.
28. Richardson S, Lawrence K, Schoenthaler AM, Mann D. A framework for digital health equity. NPJ Digit Med. 2022;5:119. https://doi.org/10.1038/s41746-022-00663-0.
29. Salud. (n.d.). GBH. Retrieved April 21, 2025, from https://www.wgbh.org/salud
30. Salud, GBH's New Health Podcast for Spanish-Speaking Audiences. (2022, November 28). GBH. https://www.wgbh.org/foundation/highlights/2022-11-28/salud-gbhs-new-health-podcast-for-spanish-speaking-audiences
31. Semakula D, Nsangi A, Oxman AD, Oxman M, Austvoll-Dahlgren A, Rosenbaum S, Morelli A, Glenton C, Lewin S, Kaseje M, Chalmers I, Fretheim A, Kristoffersen DT, Sewankambo NK. Effects of the informed health choices podcast on the ability of parents of primary school children in Uganda to assess claims about treatment effects: a randomised controlled trial. Lancet. 2017;390(10092):389–98. https://doi.org/10.1016/S0140-6736(17)31225-4.
32. Shapiro-Mendoza CK, Woodworth KR, Cottengim CR, Erck Lambert AB, Harvey EM, Monsour M, Parks SE, Barfield WD. Sudden unexpected infant deaths: 2015–2020. Pediatrics. 2023;151(4):e2022058820. https://doi.org/10.1542/peds.2022-058820.
33. Shearer E (2023, April 25). Black U.S. podcast listeners choose distinct topics, have different reasons for listening than other groups. Pew Research Center. https://www.pewresearch.org/short-reads/2023/04/25/black-u-s-podcast-listeners-choose-distinct-topics-have-different-reasons-for-listening-than-other-groups/
34. Shen MJ, Peterson EB, Costas-Muñiz R, Hernandez MH, Jewell ST, Matsoukas K, Bylund CL. The effects of race and racial concordance on patient-physician communication: a systematic review of the literature. J Racial Ethn Health Disparities. 2018;5(1):117–40. https://doi.org/10.1007/s40615-017-0350-4.
35. Sieck CJ, Sheon A, Ancker JS, Castek J, Callahan B, Siefer A. Digital inclusion as a social determinant of health. NPJ Digit Med. 2021;4:52. https://doi.org/10.1038/s41746-021-00413-8.
36. Snyder JE, Upton RD, Hassett TC, Lee H, Nouri Z, Dill M. Black representation in the primary care physician workforce and its association with population life expectancy and mortality rates in the US. JAMA Netw Open. 2023;6(4):e236687. https://doi.org/10.1001/jamanetworkopen.2023.6687.
37. Social Determinants of Health—Healthy People 2030 | odphp.health.gov. (n.d.). Retrieved April 7, 2025, from https://odphp.health.gov/healthypeople/priority-areas/social-determinants-health
38. Strengthening digital health literacy to empower people in the digital age. (n.d.). Retrieved April 7, 2025, from https://www.who.int/europe/news-room/events/item/2024/11/21/default-calendar/strengthening-digital-health-literacy-to-empower-people-in-the-digital-age

39. The Curbsiders—An Internal Medicine Podcast. (n.d.). The Curbsiders—An Internal Medicine Podcast. Retrieved April 21, 2025, from https://thecurbsiders.com
40. The Rural American Surgeon. (n.d.). The Rural American Surgeon. Retrieved April 7, 2025, from https://www.theruralamericansurgeon.com
41. Tran P, Tran L, Tran L. Impact of rurality on diabetes screening in the US. BMC Public Health. 2019;19(1):1190. https://doi.org/10.1186/s12889-019-7491-9.
42. van Kessel R, Wong BLH, Clemens T, Brand H. Digital health literacy as a super determinant of health: more than simply the sum of its parts. Internet Interv. 2022;27:100500. https://doi.org/10.1016/j.invent.2022.100500.
43. Van Niekerk L, Topp SM, Pasternak N, Mackey TK, Garcia P, Binagwaho A, Aslanyan G. Podcasts as a tool to disrupt knowledge hierarchies and silos to decolonize global health. Nat Med. 2024;30(5):1227–8. https://doi.org/10.1038/s41591-024-02859-1.
44. Viswanath K, Ackerson LK. Race, ethnicity, language, social class, and health communication inequalities: a nationally-representative cross-sectional study. PLoS One. 2011;6(1):e14550. https://doi.org/10.1371/journal.pone.0014550.
45. Woodward EN, Matthieu MM, Uchendu US, Rogal S, Kirchner JE. The health equity implementation framework: proposal and preliminary study of hepatitis C virus treatment. Implement Sci. 2019;14(1):26. https://doi.org/10.1186/s13012-019-0861-y.

Chapter 14
Overcoming Podcast Challenges

Christopher Chiu

Introduction

Medical education podcasting has experienced unprecedented growth over the past two decades. Kelly et al. [1] in their study published in Academic Medicine documented the emergence of podcasting as a predominant source for resident education. This trend is further substantiated by Cadogan et al. [2] which demonstrated a remarkable progression from a single podcast in 2002 to 42 distinct podcasts by 2013 just within the realm of Emergency Medicine and Critical Care alone. More recent data from Danford et al. [3], published in the Journal of American Academy of Orthopedic Surgeons, confirms this continued expansion. Their study, "Current Status of Podcasts in Orthopedic Surgery Practice and Education," documented a 1340% increase in orthopedic surgery podcasts between 2016 and 2021, a growth rate that reflects the medium's perceived value among specialists and educators alike.

With this proliferation comes a set of distinctive challenges that merit systematic examination. This chapter addresses three fundamental challenges inherent to medical education podcasting:

1. **Concerns about content currency and relevance.** As the catalog of episodes for any given podcast expands, earlier content may become outdated as clinical guidelines evolve, protocols are revised, and new pharmacological agents are introduced. This necessitates thoughtful strategies for distinguishing between time-sensitive content and that which remains perpetually relevant (often termed

C. Chiu (✉)
Division of General Internal Medicine, The Ohio State University Wexner Medical Center, Columbus, OH, USA
e-mail: christopher.chiu@osumc.edu

J. Parga-Belinkie et al. (eds.), *Podcasting for Medical Professionals*,
https://doi.org/10.1007/978-3-032-16480-3_14

"evergreen" content). Subsequent sections will explore methodologies for managing this challenge effectively.
2. **Limitations of audio-only instruction.** Many medical teaching skills have traditionally relied on visual demonstration. Dermatological assessments, procedural techniques, and anatomical concepts present difficulties in this regard. This chapter will examine approaches to overcome these constraints through innovative descriptive techniques and complementary resources.
3. **Variability in guest presentation skills.** Not all subject matter experts possess natural communication abilities that translate effectively to the podcast medium. This section will explore pre-interview preparation protocols, interview facilitation techniques, and post-production strategies to enhance the educational value of such interactions.

This chapter aims to provide evidence-based, practical solutions to these challenges by examining established practices, emergent technologies, and the integration of complementary educational modalities. By addressing these challenges systematically, medical education podcasters can enhance the efficacy, longevity, and impact of their content, ultimately improving learning outcomes for healthcare professionals and, by extension, patient care.

Challenge 1: Maintaining Relevant Content

There are many ways in which different podcasts may approach the identification of outdated content and ensure the episodes they produce remain current. Examining the archive of previously released episodes and considering future content based on the core listenership will help podcast producers determine clinical relevance.

Team-Based and Crowdsourced Content Development

Productions benefit from soliciting ideas from a diverse group of contributors. This works to enhance content relevance by pooling perspectives. Ideally a production would have representation from various educational stages, ranging from high school education to residency training, and junior faculty to senior career faculty positions. This multi-layered opinion gathering are an important component of the production process at *The Cribsiders*, which ensures that our episodes are able to reflect diverse clinical experiences, educational needs, and perspectives.

Aside from cultivating divergent viewpoints from the production team, maintaining a presence in the digital domain and on social media platforms facilitates continuous feedback from listeners. Listeners will also come from a range of backgrounds and can give valuable feedback regarding preferred episodes, content suggestions, and guest recommendations. This direct audience engagement serves as a valuable mechanism for content creation and relevance assessment. Social media platforms provide real-time feedback channels where listeners can flag potentially outdated information or request updates on previous topics. Establishing dedicated hashtags or regular "request for update" posts can formalize this process inviting commentary and fostering community.

Systematic Content Evaluation

Another approach to ensuring content currency involves evaluating the curricular comprehensiveness of existing episodes against established board review content for the relevant medical specialty. For example, the *Cribsiders*, a pediatric podcast, has conducted and published reviews comparing their content (and other pediatric podcasts) against the pediatric board content domains obtained from the American Board of Pediatrics website [4]. This type of retrospective analysis helps identify content gaps and informs future episode planning.

Staying abreast of current guidelines, protocols, and medications as they evolve in clinical practice provides another mechanism for identifying relevant content. As healthcare professionals maintain currency in their clinical work, they naturally encounter emerging guidelines, updated protocols, and novel therapeutic agents that may serve as topics for future episodes.

Tiered Content Classification Systems

Implementing a structured classification system enables both producers and listeners to better understand the expected longevity and update requirements for different types of content. Content can be conceptualized beyond simple "evergreen" versus "time-sensitive" categorizations:

- **Core knowledge.** Episodes focusing on fundamental pathophysiology typically require minimal updating as the underlying science changes slowly. These episodes can also be tagged as "Fundamentals" or "Foundations" series.
- **Practice guidelines.** This content requires regular updating as clinical recommendations evolve. These episodes benefit from explicit labeling with guideline edition numbers or years to clarify the currency of information.
- **Emerging evidence.** These episodes should be clearly framed as presenting preliminary information subject to revision. These might also be designated as part of a "Frontiers" or "Emerging Research" series.
- **Expert opinion.** This content should be distinguished from consensus guidelines, perhaps through a dedicated interview series explicitly acknowledging the perspective being presented.

Content Updating Rituals

Creating predictable patterns of content revision helps set appropriate listener expectations and establishes a framework for keeping content current:

Let's use an internal medical podcast called *The Curbsiders* as an example. This podcast has a "Hotcake Series" which exemplifies how a dedicated episode format can efficiently address evolving topics [5]. The "Hotcake Series" allows the producers and hosts to systematically introduce and review articles and studies with critical analysis. This approach creates a recognizable framework for listeners to expect updated information on rapidly changing subjects as a type of "Journal Club."

"Journal Club" formats discuss new evidence that confirms or challenges previous episodes and creates opportunities for nuanced discussion of evolving evidence. This format acknowledges the iterative nature of medical knowledge while maintaining scientific rigor. NephJC's Freely Filtered Podcast and PHM from Pittsburgh have great examples of these types of show [6, 7].

Lastly, annual "update" episodes revisiting high-impact topics from previous years provide a systematic approach to content currency. These episodes can explicitly reference original content while highlighting changes in understanding or practice.

CME Requirements as Structural Framework

For podcasts seeking continuing medical education (CME) accreditation, the Accreditation Council for Continuing Medical Education mandates producers review enduring materials at least once every three years, or more frequently if indicated by new scientific developments [8]. This requirement provides a structural framework for revisiting core topics and serves as a strategy for scheduling reruns of classic episodes.

In adult medicine, this might involve producing new episodes on hypertension or hyperlipidemia, evergreen topics that require periodic updates to reflect new medications or guidelines. Audience requests for updates on previous episodes may necessitate more specialized content focusing on advanced management strategies, such as next-line medications gaining acceptance in general practice.

When significant guideline changes occur that do not warrant reviewing core pathophysiology but focus exclusively on new recommendations, which may be sufficiently complex to constitute an entire episode, an update format may be most appropriate.

Digital Management of Outdated Content

As content is updated or rerun, podcast producers should consider either archiving or annotating outdated episodes on their website or distribution platform. This practice ensures that listeners accessing the back catalog receive appropriate context regarding the currency of the information presented.

Digital tagging systems can automatically flag older episodes with production dates or update status, helping listeners quickly assess content currency. Additionally, linking related episodes in series (original content and subsequent updates) creates clear pathways for listeners to access the most current information.

Challenge 2: Teaching Visual and Procedural Skills through Audio

The fundamental challenge of teaching visual or procedural content through an audio medium represents what might be considered "the elephant in the room" in medical education podcasting. Episodes on many different podcasts have necessitated sophisticated verbal descriptions of visual elements such as rashes or other physical findings.

This limitation, however, offers an unexpected pedagogical benefit: it requires clinicians to develop and refine their descriptive language skills, an essential capability in clinical practice. Clinicians must routinely describe their visual observations, whether documenting a rash or communicating visual findings to colleagues. Therefore, the constraint of audio-only presentation can enhance these vital communication skills.

Structured Approaches to Visual Description

Implementing a standardized descriptive approach significantly enhances listener comprehension. Dermatologic skin findings make a good example of a visual diagnosis translated to an audio format. Effective podcasters may utilize a systematic framework that includes:

- **Primary morphology** (macule, papule, vesicle, etc.)
- **Secondary features** (scaling, crusting, erosion)
- **Distribution pattern** (symmetric, asymmetric, localized, generalized)
- **Color characteristics and variations** (blanching, central clearing)
- **Border qualities** (well-defined, irregular, target-like)
- **Associated features** (pruritus, tenderness, contextual symptoms)

This structured approach mirrors the language clinicians should use in documentation and interprofessional communication, reinforcing valuable clinical skills while compensating for the absence of visual information.

Translating Procedures

Teaching procedures presents unique challenges in audio format, particularly for techniques involving three-dimensional movements. An example of this is point-of-care ultrasound (POCUS) instruction, where terminology like "scan" and "sweep" require precise understanding of probe manipulation. Effective podcasters develop specific techniques for translating these movements:

- **Orienting listeners** (anatomical landmarks, planes of the body)
- **Directional language** (precise reference points)
- **Comparing movements** (describing familiar everyday actions)
- **Specifying the degrees and extent of movement**
- **Describing expected changes** in visualization as movements occur

The *Ultrasound GEL* (Gathering Evidence from the Literature) podcast exemplifies an effective approach to teaching POCUS through audio [9]. Rather than attempting to describe complete procedural techniques, the podcast focuses on the evidence basis for ultrasound interventions and the clinical reasoning behind different approaches. This strategy emphasizes the "why" behind techniques, creating a cognitive framework that listeners can later apply when learning the visual and tactile components through hands-on training.

Using Analogies and Reference Points

Effective preparation with guests before recording is crucial to help listeners visualize complex visual elements. For example with dermatologic descriptions, a guest might describe the dermatomal distribution of herpes zoster as resembling "a sash draped across the torso," or with POCUS instruction, probe movements can be explained as "sweeping a flashlight across a room," providing a relatable reference point for understanding directional scanning techniques. These comparative descriptions create mental images that bridge the gap between audio description and visual understanding.

Supplementary Resources

Beyond verbal techniques, supplementary resources significantly enhance the educational value of visually challenging topics. Most podcasts maintain show notes that can incorporate appropriately credited images, diagrams, or links to complementary resources such as research studies or educational websites.

When including visual elements, content creators must carefully navigate copyright and patient privacy considerations. Dr. Avital O'Glasser's principle of "post the pearl, not the patient" provides valuable guidance [10]. This decouples the learning points from patient scenarios. The approach emphasizes sharing learning points from cases while meticulously avoiding potentially identifying information. In the digital era, seemingly de-identified cases can sometimes be reconstructed when various information elements are combined, particularly if listeners are familiar with the case description.

The AMA Journal of Ethics paper by Crane et al. outlines several important factors to consider when sharing visual content [11]:

1. **Timing:** Publication of visual elements in show notes should be delayed from the actual clinical encounter to reduce identifiability.
2. **Patient details:** These should be strictly limited, recognizing that the audience includes healthcare professionals who may be able to identify cases if given too much information.

Multimedia Approaches

Multimedia approaches offer additional solutions to the visual limitations of audio podcasting. With video platforms becoming increasingly popular for podcast distribution, incorporating video components provides a direct avenue for demonstrating visual elements. *The Curbsiders* again as an example has created companion video content for physical examination skills such as knee and shoulder examinations, which are posted separately to their YouTube platform [12].

Other visual content that may supplement audio discussions includes electrocardiograms and point-of-care ultrasound (POCUS) images. One effective strategy involves sharing links to established educational resources that have already addressed privacy and copyright concerns. Examples include The POCUS Atlas [13] for ultrasound imaging or PhysicalDiagnosisPDX [14] for physical examination skills which are resources that are freely accessible and have addressed HIPAA compliance issues.

By implementing these strategies, audio podcast creators can effectively overcome the inherent limitations of audio-only formats when teaching content that traditionally relies on visual demonstration or procedural instruction.

Challenge 3: Coaching Guests

The challenge of producing a dynamic conversation begins at the pre-interview or even pre-guest selection stage. For podcasts that utilize guests, the initial selection process represents a critical opportunity to enhance episode quality.

Pre-interview and Guest Selection Process

Identifying potential guests who have demonstrated dynamic speaking abilities, whether through personal observation of their presentations or recommendations from trusted colleagues who have heard them speak, provides a solid foundation for engaging content. This preliminary screening can significantly increase the likelihood of recording a compelling episode.

Guest Assessment Strategies

Podcast producers can implement systematic approaches to guest assessment prior to extending invitations:

- **Reviewing** previous podcast appearances or recorded presentations by potential guests
- **Consulting** with colleagues who have worked with or been taught by the prospective guest
- **Conducting brief pre-interview conversations** to gauge communication style and rapport
- **Observing teaching evaluations** when available, particularly for academic physicians

Preparation Framework

Once a guest has been identified, thorough research and preparation of a structured interview format aligned with the guest's comfort level will facilitate a more fluid discussion during recording. Many successful podcasts utilize collaborative platforms such as Google Docs or Dropbox to share interview questions with guests well in advance of recording sessions. This approach allows guests to prepare thoughtfully and reduces anxiety related to the recording process.

A comprehensive preparation framework includes:

- **Detailed biographical research** to identify the guest's specific areas of expertise and professional experiences
- **Customized question development** that aligns with the guest's published work or clinical focus
- **Clear communication** about technical requirements and recording logistics
- **Explicit discussion** of the podcast's tone, audience, and educational objectives

Anxiety Reduction Techniques

Even highly knowledgeable experts who can discuss their subject matter extensively may experience hesitation during recording. When sessions are not recorded for live broadcast, reassuring guests about the editing process and explicitly giving them permission to restate or refine their responses can alleviate pressure. In this way podcasting is a very forgiving medium. Additionally, allowing guests ample time to reflect before responding to questions often yields more thoughtful and articulate answers.

Specific strategies for reducing guest anxiety include:

- **Conducting technical checks ("sound checks")** well before content recording begins to address potential distractions
- **Emphasis conversation.** Explain pauses, reflection time, and restarts are normal and expected and allow for connection with listeners.
- **Sharing example episodes** that demonstrate how the final product will sound
- **Providing a "safe word" or signal** that guests can use to indicate when they would like to restart an answer
- **Describe the editing process** so guests know their answers can be edited and that the goal is to make them sound professional and knowledgeable on the subject matter.
- **Start with Easy Questions.** introductory "softball" questions that help establish rapport, and can effectively help guests relax before addressing more complex topics.
- **Build Rapport.** Allow time before recording to get to know the guest. This is often referred to as a "warm up" period. Ask questions about their personal interests or experiences unrelated to the medical topic. These exchanges may or may not make the final edit, but they can establish a personable connection before delving into complex clinical content.

Interview Management Techniques

Over time, hosts develop sophisticated interview management techniques that enhance guest engagement. These skills, while partly acquired through experience, include three key approaches: conversation steering frameworks, real-time adaptation, and host knowledge as a foundation for discussion.

Conversation Steering Frameworks

Conversation steering represents a fundamental skill. While sharing the interview structure with guests in advance helps maintain focus, hosts must recognize discussions may naturally evolve in unanticipated directions. The ability to be flexible, adjust questioning sequences, and pursue emergent threads often results in more authentic and engaging content.

Effective hosts employ specific steering techniques:

- **"Signposting" transitions** between topics to help guests recognize shifts in content focus
- **Summarizing complex responses** to confirm understanding before progressing
- **Using directed follow-up questions** to explore areas where the guest demonstrates enthusiasm
- **Employing the "yes, and" approach** from improvisational techniques to build upon guest responses

Real-Time Adaptation

Taking strategic "time-outs" during recording sessions to consult with co-hosts about the conversation's direction allows for real-time adjustments to ensure alignment with the episode's objectives. Some podcasts have developed subtle signals among co-hosts to indicate when a conversation requires redirection or when a particularly valuable thread should be pursued further.

Host Knowledge as Foundation

Perhaps most critically, thorough topic preparation by the host is essential. A common misconception holds that hosts need minimal subject knowledge because guests will provide all necessary information. In reality when hosts approach the guest's level of expertise, they can pose more insightful questions and guide the conversation more effectively toward the envisioned content. Thus, the host's knowledge serves as a crucial safety net ensuring episode quality even when guest dynamics present challenges.

The depth of host preparation manifests in several ways:

- The ability to ask **sophisticated follow-up questions** that demonstrate genuine engagement
- Capacity to **translate complex concepts** into accessible language for listeners
- Recognition of **opportunities to connect guest expertise** with previously covered topics
- Confidence to **redirect conversations** when they veer from educational objectives

Post-production Solutions

When preparation, pre-interview strategies, and interview management techniques still result in a less dynamic discussion, post-production solutions offer additional remediation options. Skilled editing can significantly improve flow, particularly with guests whose responses tend to meander. Adding contextual elements and clarifications through post-production dialogue from hosts or other contributors can enhance comprehensibility and engagement.

Editorial Techniques

Specific editorial approaches include:

- **Removing false starts and verbal fillers** (ie. umms, ahhs, and use of the word like) that might distract from substantive content
- **Restructuring conversation sequences** to create more logical progression of ideas
- **Shortening lengthy explanations** while preserving essential teaching points
- **Adding transition elements** between conceptually related but temporally separated discussions

Host Commentary Integration

Many medical education podcasts enhance less dynamic guest segments by interspersing host commentary:

- **Brief explanations or simplifications** following complex guest responses
- **Clinical application examples** that illustrate abstract concepts in clinical contexts
- **Connections to current guidelines or standard practices** that contextualize guest expertise
- **Summary statements** to highlight key takeaways from detailed discussions

Technical Enhancements

Audio production techniques can also enhance engagement:

- **Normalization of audio levels** to ensure guest contributions have equivalent presence
- Strategic use of **music or sound elements** to maintain listener attention during transitions
- **Intentional pauses or segment breaks** to manage cognitive load
- Implementation of **varied pacing** to maintain listener engagement

Balancing Authenticity and Engagement

Throughout this process, balancing authentic discussion with audience engagement remains paramount. Some of the most successful episodes may venture into unexpected territory based on guest expertise, creating content superior to what was initially envisioned.

When evaluating this balance, podcast producers might consider:

- The **educational value** of the content versus its entertainment quality
- The degree to which editing **preserves the guest's authentic voice** and perspective
- Opportunities for **follow-up episodes or supplementary content** to address areas where detailed exploration was limited
- **Feedback mechanisms** that allow listeners to indicate topics requiring additional clarification (as described above)

By implementing these comprehensive strategies across pre-interview, interview, and post-production phases, medical education podcasters can consistently produce engaging, valuable content even when working with less naturally dynamic guests.

The Evolving Landscape of Medical Education Podcasting

The rapid growth of medical education podcasting reflects the medium's capacity to deliver accessible, engaging, and clinically relevant content to healthcare professionals. Throughout this chapter, we have examined three fundamental challenges podcast creators encounter: maintaining relevant content, teaching visual and procedural skills via audio, and engaging less dynamic guests. The strategies outlined for addressing these challenges demonstrate that thoughtful planning, innovative approaches, and technological integration can effectively overcome the medium's inherent limitations.

As we look toward the future, several developments suggest that medical education podcasting will continue its evolution as a central component of the continuing education landscape. Emerging technologies will increasingly address the medium's current limitations, while changing consumption patterns will shape content development.

Technological Integration and Innovation

The boundaries between podcast platforms and other digital learning environments continue to blur as technological integration accelerates. Interactive podcast interfaces now enable synchronized access to visual content, reference materials, and assessment tools, creating more comprehensive educational experiences.

Perhaps most transformative is the integration of artificial intelligence into medical education podcasting workflows. AI applications now support hosts in multiple critical areas:

- **Evidence Surveillance:** AI-powered literature monitoring tools continuously scan medical journals, clinical guidelines, and research publications to identify emerging evidence relevant to previous podcast topics. This enables hosts to stay abreast of developments that might necessitate content updates without manual review of thousands of publications.
- **Content Preparation Assistance:** Advanced natural language processing systems assist hosts in synthesizing complex clinical literature, identifying key controversies, and formulating nuanced discussion points. This significantly reduces preparation time while ensuring comprehensive topic coverage.
- **Automated Content Analysis:** Machine learning algorithms can now analyze podcast archives to identify potentially outdated medical information, suggest appropriate update intervals based on the rate of evidence evolution in particular fields, and even generate draft supplementary resources for listener reference.

These AI integrations address the fundamental challenge of maintaining relevant, evidence-based content in a rapidly evolving medical landscape. By leveraging these technologies, podcast producers can focus more attention on effective communication and engaging presentation while ensuring underlying content remains scientifically current. As part of this process, due diligence requires verifying AI-generated content against primary sources to mitigate the risk of hallucinations or inaccuracies, ensuring that the final educational product remains trustworthy and evidence-based.

Changing Patterns of Consumption and Engagement

Listener behavior continues to evolve from passive consumption toward active engagement. Analytics reveal increasingly purposeful listening patterns, with healthcare professionals setting aside dedicated time for podcast education rather than relegating it to background listening during other activities. This shift enables podcasters to develop more complex, detailed content without sacrificing audience engagement.

This active engagement is evident in the growing utilization of platform-specific interactive features. Comment sections on YouTube can feature clinical discussions, with some listeners posing follow-up questions, sharing relevant clinical experiences, or occasionally linking to supporting or contradictory evidence. The Curbsiders podcast, for instance, sometimes sees comments on YouTube that extend the educational conversation beyond the episode itself, with clinicians commenting on aspects of guidelines or sharing implementation strategies from their institutions. Additionally, some podcast platforms now offer enhanced listening experiences through episode ratings, reviews, and discussion forums that allow listeners to engage with content after listening, further developing the educational community around medical podcasts.

The platform landscape for medical education podcasting is also undergoing significant transformation. Video platforms, particularly YouTube, are outpacing traditional audio-only platforms like Spotify and Apple Podcasts in terms of educational content consumption [15]. This shift toward visual platforms reflects listeners' desire for multimodal learning experiences that address the challenges of teaching visual or procedural skills. Medical education podcasters increasingly produce "vodcasts" that maintain audio quality while incorporating visual elements such as slides, anatomical illustrations, clinical images, and procedural demonstrations when appropriate (see Sheriff of Sodium) [16]. This evolution expands the educational possibilities while maintaining the convenience that initially attracted audiences to the podcast format.

Furthermore, the social dimension of podcast learning is expanding beyond traditional platforms into diverse digital spaces. While engagement on X (formerly Twitter) and Facebook remains common, discussions are increasingly migrating to platforms like Reddit, where dedicated subreddits for medical specialties host in-depth conversations about podcast content. More significantly, closed community spaces are emerging as vital hubs for deeper educational engagement. Discord servers dedicated to specific medical podcasts allow for real-time discussion and knowledge exchange between listeners and sometimes podcast creators themselves. Subscription-based platforms like Patreon are evolving beyond simple funding mechanisms to become exclusive educational communities where podcasters share additional resources, respond to listener questions, and facilitate focused discussions away from the noise of public social media.

These specialized digital communities offer several advantages over public platforms: they allow for more candid clinical discussions with appropriate privacy, create space for nuanced exploration of complex topics, and foster professional relationships among listeners with shared interests. Medical education podcasters increasingly leverage these spaces to gather feedback, test content ideas, and build sustained educational communities that extend the impact of their audio content. This evolution transforms what began as a solitary learning activity into a collaborative educational experience with meaningful professional connections.

Conclusion

The challenges discussed in this chapter, while significant, have inspired innovative solutions that enhance the medium's educational potential. As technologies advance and consumption patterns evolve, podcasting will continue to develop as a sophisticated educational modality with unique advantages for healthcare professionals.

The success of medical education podcasting ultimately rests not on technological capabilities but on the thoughtful application of educational principles to this accessible medium. By addressing content currency, visual limitations, and interview dynamics systematically, podcast creators can produce educational experiences that meaningfully impact clinical knowledge, reasoning, and practice.

As we look toward the future, the collaborative spirit that characterizes the medical podcasting community will continue to drive innovation and excellence in this evolving medium. The shared commitment to enhancing healthcare education through accessible, engaging content ensures medical education podcasting will remain at the forefront of continuing professional development for years to come.

References

1. https://pubmed.ncbi.nlm.nih.gov/34935729/
2. https://pubmed.ncbi.nlm.nih.gov/24554447/
3. https://pubmed.ncbi.nlm.nih.gov/34736272/
4. Ledingham L, Jacob B, Chiu C. Plugged. In: Curricular comprehensiveness of popular pediatric medical podcasts. Honolulu: 2025 Pediatric Academic Societies; April 24, 2025.
5. https://thecurbsiders.com/tag/hotcakes
6. https://www.nephjc.com/freelyfiltered
7. https://pedhospmed.libsyn.com/website
8. https://accme.org/rule/content-validity-of-enduring-materials/
9. https://www.ultrasoundgel.org/
10. https://x.com/aoglasser/status/1236053604080873473
11. https://pubmed.ncbi.nlm.nih.gov/27550566/
12. https://www.youtube.com/playlist?list=PL5oEcyJ-glk5Aac2vD2imCGYYTteq9eTB
13. https://www.thepocusatlas.com/
14. https://physicaldiagnosispdx.com/
15. https://www.westwoodone.com/blog/2024/07/08/youtubes-growth-as-a-podcast-power-player-revealed-in-cumulus-media-and-signal-hill-insights-podcast-download-spring-2024-report/
16. https://youtube.com/@sheriffofsodium

Chapter 15
The Future of Medical Podcasting

Jeffrey Goddard

Introduction

In the immortal words of the baseball player, Yogi Berra, "it is difficult to make predictions, especially about the future." Looking back over the last 100 years, seismic shifts in technology have been entirely unforeseeable. It is with great humility, then, that an attempt will be made in this chapter to suggest the future of medical podcasting. These predictions are not unfounded. They are based on emerging trends that show the most promise for future growth and adaptation. While nothing in the future is set in stone, reasonable predictions can and must be made to make decisions on how to proceed. Indeed, some of these predictions are based on emerging trends that we see today but for which we have not yet realized the full potential.

The Convergence of Audio and Visual Content

While many will continue to prefer content that can be enjoyed entirely through their headphones, there will be a growing demand for creators who are willing to create visual content to compliment the audio experience. Splicing video with audio can provide a more engaging visual experience and may become more necessary in the future.

There is, and will likely continue to be, a significant market for content creators who host their podcast conversations in front of a camera, with minimal video editing—giving viewers a behind-the-scenes view of the podcasting milieu. The

J. Goddard (✉)
University of Iowa Carver College of Medicine, Iowa City, Iowa, USA
e-mail: jeffrey-goddard@uiowa.edu

J. Parga-Belinkie et al. (eds.), *Podcasting for Medical Professionals*,
https://doi.org/10.1007/978-3-032-16480-3_15

simplicity of these videos works because the most engaging content these creators can offer is their own personality and presence.

The continued development of technologies such as AI will make it possible to do more with less, as the previous chapter on AI has shown. Few doctors are graphic artists or confident script writers and editing can be a Sisyphean task. But as AI improves, more of this work can be automated, allowing creators to focus on the most important aspect of their podcast, and the part to which they are most qualified to address: the medical content itself.

The Audio-Visual Decision: Practical Considerations

Why the Market Is Shifting Toward Visual

The podcast market is increasingly embracing visual components for several practical reasons. First, platform algorithms—particularly on YouTube—tend to favor video content, giving greater visibility to creators who incorporate visual elements. This extends the reach of a podcast significantly with relatively little investment. Second, audience data consistently shows longer engagement times with visual content, and YouTube is leading the pack in podcast listens according to Edison Research [1].

For medical content specifically, visualization addresses a fundamental challenge: medical concepts and procedures often require visual explanation. Whether demonstrating physical exam techniques, explaining anatomical relationships, or reviewing imaging studies, visual elements can significantly enhance comprehension [2–4]. Graphics need not be complex or novel, but may include a graphic from a paper being discussed or an image of a CT scan relevant to the topic of the episode. Audiences will appreciate not having to go to the show notes for everything talked about in an episode.

The rise of short-form content platforms has also accelerated this shift. TikTok, Instagram Reels, and YouTube Shorts have created enormous audiences accustomed to consuming educational content in visual formats. Medical podcasters who create visual content can repurpose segments for these platforms, exponentially increasing their reach and driving new listeners to their full-length episodes. The goal is not necessarily to master the short form, but rather to feed back into full length podcast episodes.

Making the Decision: Audio-Only Versus Visual

For a new medical podcaster, here's a practical decision framework:

Choose audio-only if:

- Your content focuses primarily on interviews, discussions, or narrative storytelling
- You have limited time and technical resources for production
- Your target audience consists mainly of busy clinicians who listen during commutes
- You plan to cover sensitive or controversial topics where video might inhibit guest openness
- You plan to discuss topics or conditions that may be unsettling for lay audiences to see visually, such as necrosis.

Add visual components if:

- Your content regularly involves explaining procedures, physical findings, or imaging
- You aim to reach students and trainees who often use multiple learning modalities
- You want to maximize content repurposing for growth on social platforms
- You have the time, equipment, or team to manage video production
- Your personality and presentation style are particularly engaging on camera

Many successful medical podcasters begin with audio-only and gradually incorporate visual elements as they build their audience and production capabilities. While podcast audiences of the future will be gravitating more to visual content, there will always be a place for purely audio podcasts. Remember that trends can inform but needn't drive your every decision.

Short-Form Content Revolution

Medical podcasting and short-form video might initially seem like different worlds, or at least different markets—one built around in-depth conversations that often span an hour or more, the other centered on quick, attention-grabbing clips measured in seconds. Yet for the strategic medical podcaster, these formats represent complementary components of a cohesive content strategy rather than competing approaches. The future will see greater and greater integration of these two worlds.

A whole generation has gotten their information and entertainment in one-to-five-minute chunks on platforms such as Snapchat, TikTok, and Instagram Reels. Social media platforms require creators to formulate a cohesive yet succinct message in a short video format. This format is often much more organic than long form videos because the short video format allows clinicians to showcase their personality and converse with, rather than lecture, their audience.

The connection between podcasting and short-form content is fundamentally about audience building and content maximization. Podcasts contain dozens of insightful moments, compelling explanations, and memorable analogies that can stand alone as powerful short-form content. By extracting and repurposing these moments, you transform a single podcast episode into multiple entry points for new listeners. It is reasonable to consider these as a spin on the original, becoming their own subsidiary brand of content that might have their own audience apart from the core podcast following.

The downsides must be understood: less nuance fits in a 5-minute video than a full podcast episode. This often leads to several follow up videos clarifying and threading challenging concepts delicately. Depending on the platform, these videos may not be easily linked to one another, leaving both the creator and the consumer feeling disjointed while trying to find a full series. In the future, the linkage between podcasts and short-form social content will likely be easier, allowing audiences to navigate between both mediums seamlessly.

Regardless how one might feel about the short-form format, it seems only to be gaining popularity. The future of any given platform cannot be confidently predicted, but the format itself will be part of the future landscape of medical information sharing.

Short-Form Content: A Practical Strategy for Medical Podcasters

For the practical podcaster, short-form video serves several specific functions:

1. Audience Acquisition: Short videos act as discovery tools, introducing your content to people who would never seek out a full-length medical podcast. When someone encounters your 60-second explanation of hypertension guidelines on TikTok, they may follow the link to your full episode on treatment approaches.
2. Content Atomization: A one-hour podcast typically contains 7–10 distinct educational points that can each become standalone short videos, multiplying your content output without requiring entirely new material.
3. Platform Diversification: Many listeners discover podcasts not through podcast apps but via social media. A short-form video strategy ensures your content appears where potential listeners already spend their time.
4. Algorithmic Advantage: Short-form platforms often provide greater organic reach than podcast directories. A 90-second clip might reach tens of thousands of viewers on Instagram Reels, compared to the few hundred who might organically discover your podcast episode.
5. Topic Testing: Before committing to a full episode on a specific medical topic, you can gauge interest by posting short-form content on the subject and measuring engagement.

Educational Applications

Podcasts are already gaining a positive reputation as medical education across the continuum from pre-med to experienced clinicians and this will only continue as time goes on.

The market is far from saturated, and there remains a significant need for medical experts in every discipline to share their knowledge. The future will yield not only opportunity but obligation for providers to effectively communicate their expertise. In turn, the podcast market will provide better crafted, masterclass messaging that can be easily accessed by all. Learners have a dire need for voices that they can trust at a time when misinformation is pervasive, as well as episodes that distill complex concepts and frontier science into digestible chunks in a world with fast-paced changes in research impacting clinical practice.

If medical professionals and learners are demanding the democratization of knowledge, the public at large is doing so with much more force. Visits to their healthcare provider often leave patients with unanswered question and they turn to online resources for answers and explanations. The future of medical podcasting for patients is to be able to find the episode or series that addresses their questions about their new diagnosis. Providers will be able to save their favorite podcast episodes and prescribe them to patients in clinic. The prescription of knowledge to individualize education for patients beyond what clinicians can offer in the clinic extends the educational impact of the clinical encounter. Content can be as specific to their cultural background and/or language, truly meeting them where they are, even when we as providers are not always able to effectively do so.

Ensuring Content Quality

The future of medical podcasting will likely see more formalized quality assurance mechanisms. We might see a system where medical podcasts receive certification badges indicating they've undergone expert review, like the way journals are indexed in PubMed. These certifications could signal to listeners—whether they're patients, medical students, or providers—that the content meets established standards for accuracy and evidence-based practice.

The challenge lies in balancing rigorous quality control with the nimble, responsive nature that makes podcasting valuable. Current systems for peer-review of podcasts are labor-intensive and that slow pace does not fit with the podcasting world. Future systems will need to find the balance of verifiable credibility and efficiency, perhaps through post-publication peer review, listener feedback mechanisms, AI-drive peer review rubrics, or tiered verification systems that differentiate between opinion, clinical experience, and evidence-based recommendations.

Measuring Impact

Traditional impact metrics for academic work, like citation counts or impact factors, don't translate directly to podcasting. Download numbers and subscriber counts tell only part of the story and say little about the actual effect on clinical practice or patient outcomes. The future will demand more sophisticated approaches to impact assessment.

Innovative medical podcasters are already beginning to measure knowledge retention through integrated assessment tools, tracking how content translates to clinical decision-making or influences patient behavior. These early efforts hint at more robust frameworks to come.

Future impact measurement might include:

- Knowledge transfer assessments that measure not just exposure to content but actual learning
- Behavioral change tracking among healthcare providers who regularly consume specific podcast content
- Patient outcome studies that correlate podcast-based education with health results
- Engagement quality metrics that go beyond simple listening time to measure active information processing

As podcasting becomes increasingly integrated with healthcare delivery systems, new opportunities for impact assessment will emerge. Imagine a future where an electronic health record can track which educational podcasts a patient has consumed and correlate this with their health literacy scores, medication adherence, or treatment outcomes. Such systems would provide unprecedented insight into the real-world impact of medical podcasting content. Correlating treatment decisions among clinicians and the podcasts they listen to could further our efforts in evidence-based medicine.

The medical podcasters of tomorrow will need to build assessment into their content strategy from the beginning—not as an afterthought but as a core component of their educational mission.

Institutional Adoption and Integration

Institutional podcasts, which bring together many voices from an institution and are accessible to patients and providers, will serve multiple purposes: patient education, marketing, community outreach, and internal professional development. By creating branded podcast content, healthcare systems can ensure they extend their educational reach far beyond their physical walls. This will become an esteemed achievement of institutions and something that brings notoriety to the institution's reputation.

EHR and Clinical Workflow Integration

The next frontier for medical podcasting lies in deeper integration with clinical workflows and electronic health records. Future systems might include:

- Patient portal integration allowing seamless access to recommended medical podcasts
- Documentation tools that track which educational content patients have consumed, when, if they completed it, etc.
- Automated suggestions for relevant podcast content, based on clinical documentation, that both the provider and patient can see
- Patient-reported outcome measures linked to podcast-based education
- Secure discussion forums where patients can engage with content alongside their care teams

This kind of integration addresses one of the current limitations of medical podcasting: the disconnect between content consumption and clinical care. When podcasts become part of the official medical record, both patients and providers can reference shared information, creating common ground for discussions during appointments.

Global Perspectives and Access

The future of medical podcasting extends far beyond the English-speaking, high-resource settings where the medium first flourished. As healthcare challenges transcend borders, so too must medical education and communication. The coming decade will likely witness a paradigm shift toward truly global medical podcasting that addresses disparities in both content creation and consumption.

Breaking Down Language Barriers

Language remains one of the most significant barriers to global medical education. While English-language medical podcasts dominate the current landscape, this represents a significant limitation for most of the world's healthcare providers and patients. The integration of artificial intelligence into podcasting platforms promises to transform this reality.

Real-time AI translation and interpretation tools are already beginning to make inroads in medical podcasting. These technologies allow listeners to consume content in their preferred language while preserving the nuance and technical accuracy essential for medical communication. In the future, AI will become more accurate at translation of medical terminology, making this technology more ubiquitous and extending the reach of podcasts globally.

Addressing Infrastructure Challenges

Access limitations extend beyond language to infrastructure realities. In regions with limited internet connectivity, traditional streaming models can be prohibitively data-intensive or simply impossible. Forward-thinking medical podcasters are developing innovative solutions to these challenges.

Use of compressed audio formats and scheduled downloading will make medical education accessible despite connectivity challenges. Other programs have reimagined distribution entirely, creating podcast content that can be shared via basic mobile networks or preloaded onto devices during training sessions. The future will likely bring more sophisticated offline access solutions, potentially including community listening hubs in healthcare facilities, medical-podcast specific devices with preloaded content libraries, and mesh network distribution systems that allow content sharing without continuous internet access.

Contextualizing Content for Local Relevance

Access isn't merely about technology—it's also about relevance. Medical podcasting has historically centered Western healthcare perspectives, often failing to acknowledge resource differentials or cultural contexts that influence medical practice globally. The next generation of medical podcasters is beginning to address this through collaborative content creation models that bring together voices from diverse healthcare settings. Programs will feature rotating hosts from different countries discussing medical topics from their local perspectives, helping listeners understand both universal principles and contextual adaptation. This will allow greater dissemination of knowledge across diverse practice contexts, making it easier for providers to learn from peers how to take care of patients no matter their geography.

The ultimate vision for global medical podcasting transcends mere translation or technology—it envisions a truly democratized medium where healthcare knowledge flows multidirectionally across borders, enriching practice everywhere through diverse perspectives and contextually appropriate solutions.

Integration with Medical Education

Medical schools have approached podcasts as supplements to traditional core curriculum. However, forward-thinking institutions are now recognizing the unique advantages these platforms offer. More and more we will see podcasts integrated into pre-clinical and clerkship curriculum. Schools that lean into the democratization of medical education will see lowered costs, greater diversity in educators, and likely improved satisfaction and learning for students.

Clinical Integration and Just-in-Time Learning

Perhaps the most promising educational application lies in clinical contexts. Medical students and residents often encounter unfamiliar conditions or procedures during rotations, creating perfect "teachable moments" that traditional educational models struggle to address in real-time. In the future, podcast libraries organized by specialty, condition, or procedure will allow learners to access relevant content precisely when their motivation and need for understanding peak.

Residency programs have begun creating rotation-specific podcast playlists, with episodes carefully selected to align with the clinical conditions that residents are likely to encounter. These curated collections serve as audio companions to traditional resources like textbooks and journal articles, offering contextualized knowledge curated by rotation directors at the institutional level. In the future, standardized playlists can be developed and shared between residency programs, decreasing the burden at the local level and sharing best practices across specialties.

Faculty Development and Creation Opportunities

The integration of podcasting into medical education extends beyond consumption to creation. The University of Iowa, as an example, has a podcast created by the students. Students can host and/or produce episodes, as well as help with audio and video editing. This offers students opportunities to gain valuable experience that they will take with them into their careers. The podcast is both educational and a way to give back to the school. The University of Iowa is not the only school where students have found podcasting opportunities, though it may currently be the most robust student podcasting effort at a medical school. More schools and residency programs will likely implement similar initiatives in the future.

Future Trajectories in Medical Education

Looking ahead, I believe we should anticipate deeper integration of podcasting into formal medical education through adaptive learning systems that recommend specific episodes based on individual performance data, seamless incorporation into electronic learning portfolios, and greater recognition of podcast-based learning in competency assessments. Not only should we expect it, but we should also advocate for it. The boundaries between traditional lecture-based education and podcast-delivered content will likely continue to blur, creating hybrid models that leverage the strengths of each approach. Integration of podcasts will improve the way we deliver knowledge to the next generation of physicians.

AI and the Future

With additional AI training, clinicians will be able to write a prescription and give it to an AI to generate a full podcast episode with the voice of the creator, explaining the prescription and treatment plan to a patient. Other future applications include an AI co-host, or an AI-audience member asking real-time questions on behalf of the lay audience. In addition, AI can create visual graphics, generating images demonstrating what you are discussing, including histology slides, radiographic scans, or research graphs. Also, generative AI will be able to fact-check creators in real-time, preventing the spread of misinformation, Whatever the future holds, safely assume that to some extent AI will be a part of it.

Conclusion: The Future of Medical Podcasting

As we look toward the horizon of medical podcasting, I'm stuck on Yogi Berra's wisdom that opened this chapter. The landscape we've contemplated—from immersive technologies to global access solutions, from quality measurement frameworks to ethical considerations—represents not just possibilities but in many cases emerging realities that will shape how medical knowledge is shared and consumed. But the future often changes on a dime, and maybe little of this will come to pass. We don't know what we don't know about the technologies and trends that tomorrow brings, but we move forward with the reasonable understanding that we currently have.

The future of medical podcasting is not revolutionary but rather evolutionary-driven by creators who push boundaries while remaining grounded in the core purpose: improving healthcare through accessible education and communication.

What makes this medium particularly powerful is its inherent adaptability. Unlike traditional medical textbooks or formal curricula, podcasting can respond rapidly to emerging needs—whether that's explaining a novel pathogen during a pandemic or addressing healthcare disparities illuminated by new research. This responsiveness, coupled with increasing sophistication in production and distribution, positions medical podcasting to become not just a supplement to traditional education but a primary vehicle for knowledge dissemination in many contexts. Its democratization represents at once its greatest vulnerability and its greatest strength: everyday clinicians creating content that matters to them. In turn, podcast creators have a responsibility to uphold standards of accuracy, ethics, and quality as the medium grows in influence.

The most transformative aspect of medical podcasting's future may be its power to humanize medicine. In an era of increasing technological sophistication and specialization, the human voice—with all its warmth, nuance, and authenticity—creates connections that transcend geographical and professional boundaries. Whether discussing complex pathophysiology, sharing patient narratives, or exploring systemic challenges, podcasts remind us that medicine is fundamentally about human experience.

For those committed to advancing healthcare communication for the benefit of providers and patients alike, the invitation to participate in shaping this future, not just passively by listening to podcast, but in content creation, is present. The most exciting innovations in medical podcasting are to come. They are waiting for the next generation of medical communicators to envision and implement them.

Sources

1. https://www.edisonresearch.com/youtube-is-the-preferred-podcast-listening-service/
2. Cardoso AF, Moreli L, Braga FTMM, Vasques CI, Santos CB, Carvalho EC. Effect of a video on developing skills in undergraduate nursing students for the management of totally implantable central venous access ports. Nurse Educ Today. 2012;32(6):709–13. https://doi.org/10.1016/j.nedt.2011.09.012.
3. Holland A, Smith F, McCrossan G, Adamson E, Watt S, Penny K. Online video in clinical skills education of oral medication administration for undergraduate student nurses: a mixed methods, prospective cohort study. Nurse Educ Today. 2013;33(6):663–70. https://doi.org/10.1016/j.nedt.2012.01.006.
4. Green JL, Suresh V, Bittar P, Ledbetter L, Mithani SK, Allori A. The utilization of video technology in surgical education: a systematic review. J Surg Res. 2019;235:171–80. https://doi.org/10.1016/j.jss.2018.09.015.

Index

J. Parga-Belinkie et al. (eds.), *Podcasting for Medical Professionals*,
https://doi.org/10.1007/978-3-032-16480-3

MIX
Papier aus verantwortungsvollen Quellen
Paper from responsible sources
FSC® C105338

If you have any concerns about our products,
you can contact us on
ProductSafety@springernature.com

In case Publisher is established outside the EU,
the EU authorized representative is:
Springer Nature Customer Service Center GmbH
Europaplatz 3, 69115 Heidelberg, Germany

Printed by Libri Plureos GmbH
in Hamburg, Germany